THE GRA

The miraculous story of how th
nothing but grapes, overcame
kidney disorder. He shows how this and other diets and methods
of natural healing can be used to treat many debilitating illnesses
such as arthritis, alcoholism and stomach ulcers.

THE GRAPE CURE

A Personal Testament

Basil Shackleton

THORSONS PUBLISHING GROUP
Wellingborough, Northamptonshire

———— · ————

Rochester, Vermont

First published 1969
First published in this format 1987

British Library Cataloguing in Publication Data

Shackleton, Basil
The grape cure: a living testament.
1. Grapes — Therapeutic use
I. Title
615.8'54   RM666.G75

ISBN 0-7225-1457-3

Printed and bound in Great Britain

CONTENTS

CHAPTER ONE

THE MIRACLE

There is magic in the world—and there are miracles! Or so I believed after the remarkable cure which came to me about ten years ago—after nearly forty years of chronic illness. I was condemned to die for the want of a miracle—the only thing which could keep life in my miserable body whose throb was at its very lowest ebb.

My mind was frustrated and hope was the furthest thing within the reach of my despairing spirit. My one and only kidney harboured a nephritis—an infection which would not respond to the treatment of any of the modern wonder drugs.

Loneliness and worry added its fuel to an already desperate situation—for the body, it seemed, was on the verge of abdominal cancer—if it had not already developed that dreaded disease.

In desperation I decided to experiment on myself with a treatment I had only vaguely heard of—and about which I knew absolutely nothing. It was known as the Grape Cure. *The outcome, after twenty-three days on the treatment, was so successful that it can be likened to an absolute miracle!*

Although there was irreparable damage within my body —as a result of three major internal operations—which included the removal of my right kidney twenty-three years previously, I came through the grape treatment looking and feeling twenty years younger—*and I was completely and permanently cured!* An abscess in my only kidney had come away by its roots. My body had been freed of all toxins and subsequent pains, but far, far more important than this, at the age of fifty-three, I had recaptured the supreme joy of living. My body became charged with a new vitality. I felt radiant and whole. My mind was mellow and perfectly contented, and my spirit had become a vivid and living thing again.

The experience was a truly remarkable transformation of a sick and dying body into a fine and healthy balance again, and it proved to me, quite conclusively, that the vast majority of ailing people—whatever the nature of the illness—can be permanently cured through the medium of the ordinary table grape, with the aid, of course, of the mind and the spirit : the body itself being a self-healing organ. The chemicals in the grape are almost magical in their healing properties.

Good health is the birth-right of every human being—and every creature for that matter—but the modern way of living makes it impossible for people to achieve and maintain it without a pattern of strict, self-balanced discipline.

The remarkable chemicals in the grape offer the perfect cleansing aid to the self-healing body, and therefore perfect health to everyone. This has been proved time and again by hundreds of people who have cured themselves of varying forms of chronic illness. Because the treatment has proved itself to be so incredibly successful, I have recorded details of the whole personal experience—so that sufferers throughout the world may also benefit.

It is not sufficient for me to say, *"I lived on grapes, and grapes alone for seven weeks, and that on the twenty-third day of the treatment, an abscess came away by the roots from my one and only kidney, and that my body had completely cured itself—after all orthodox medical treatment had failed over a period of about forty years."*

Although this is exactly what did happen, this simple statement does not convey the significance, the drama or the magnitude of the experience; nor could it inspire sufferers of even the mildest illness to partake of the treatment with the absolute conviction of a cure. Nowadays, people need evidence of startling phenomena to be convinced of *bona fide* claims. To achieve this it is necessary for me to relate the whole story of my illness, from its commencement in my boyhood; as well as the pattern of unsuccessful medical treatment I had received during all those years; and finally, my fortunate discovery of the grape treatment when I was virtually on the point of death; proving that through it and balanced thought, I was restored to perfect and permanent good health—a state which is available to the vast majority of sick people who really want to get well!

CHAPTER TWO

MY ILLNESS

It all began during my school holidays. I was about twelve years old at the time. My family lived in the Matopos, near the burial place of Cecil John Rhodes—the great founder of Rhodesia. Here was a cradle of beauty—breathtaking—but in absolute contrast to the calm and lush elegance of the English countryside, with its radiations of peace and goodwill; or even the majesty of the blue-tipped mountains in the Cape of Southern Africa, as they guard and guide their rivers into the open mouths of the sea.

The beauty of the Matopos was different. The hard and cruel streak running through it blended so well with the dry, sun-baked harshness of the earth, and the shining, solid kopjies—the small jagged hills which seemed to grow out of the earth for no reason at all. Its name—THE WORLD'S VIEW —does not exaggerate the grandeur and incomparable beauty of this part of Africa.

During school holidays, with young friends as our guests, my brother and I would organise miniature safaris for the day —moving out on foot in the early morning, before the rising of the sun—having prepared our food and kit the night before. Our young minds were all agog with excitement of impending peril—for deadly poisonous snakes were abundant. Lions lurked in the long grass, and the leopard was ever alert in his places of hiding. In the evening, exhausted by the long day's trek, we would return home—but very rarely with an exciting trophy!

How wonderful is the age of youth, alive with imagination and the spirit of adventure!

The following day, charged with new and abounding energy, we would invent games, and after the intense heat of the afternoon, would all swim in the river. There, secreted in its muddy camouflage, was a peril far, far greater and certainly more dangerous than the ferocious animals or the poisonous snakes. In our ignorance and with the spirit of unfettered youth, we hurled our young bodies with great abandon and terrific splash into the still waters—for such is the urge when the sun is burning hot, and the air crisp and dry. Yes! That was the beginning of it all—the beginning of forty years of constant illness, pain, fear and frustration, *because that narrow and shallow river was the breeding ground of a scourge—a scourge, which for thousands of years has devastated the Egyptians along the banks of the Nile, as well as people of all colours in most parts of Africa.* The scourge of bilharzia, a microscopic bug with a snout like a corkscrew, which, after entering the human bladder, bores its way as far as the kidneys—breaking down the tissues and walls of the ureters—those thin connecting tubes between the kidney and the bladder—and drawing blood, the first symptoms of the disease, but the beginning of a slow and gradual process of utter destruction!

Gradually the bilharzia bug took its toll. Within a year I was the absolute victim of spasmodic attacks of renal colic—a dull, sickly and almost unbearable pain which started in the kidney and found continuity of expression through the whole length of the ureter until its reached the testicles. There would be little or no warning of an approaching attack. After an hour or so, vomiting would start. That very unpleasant state of affairs would continue for several hours—sometimes as much as five or six—on an empty stomach! What an utter contrast to the joy and happiness I had discovered in hunting and swimming. Finally, absolute exhaustion from pain and retching compelled me to accept the one thing against which my whole being instinctively rebelled—the inevitable injection of morphia! Then sleep. Blessed sleep!

The following morning I was always up and about as usual, feeling fairly fit, but for a soreness in the sensitive kidney area. These attacks went on for several years in much the same pattern. A couple every month. There was nothing which the good-hearted medical men could do, other than give synthetic relief during the actual attacks.

About five years later they became more frequent—once and sometimes twice a week. There was no rule as to which kidney was to take the burden. It seemed to oscillate from one to the other—each taking a turn as though it was a game, but, thank goodness, only one kidney had an innings at a time!

It is certainly not my wish in this narrative to talk about personal suffering as such, because as the years roll by and the roots of maturity find their destined level, it is easy to recognise that physical suffering can be a privilege. To enable me, however, to carry my story to its natural conclusion without exaggeration, I must inevitably record incidents of pain and anguish. Week in and week out for almost ten years the attacks of renal colic persisted—and then the pattern changed. After a very severe attack I passed a small stone (gravel) in the urine. It was no larger than an orange pip, and much the same shape. It looked as though it had been dipped in brown sugar. This new turn of events prompted my doctor to send me to Johannesburg for x-rays. The negative showed another small stone wedged in the right ureter between the kidney and the bladder. That meant business! The business of a major operation!!

Science has advanced so much since 1928 that an operation involving the opening of the stomach from one end to the other, to get to the ureter, is no longer necessary. However, I was prepared for surgery to remove the stone. When the operation was over, it was discovered that something had gone wrong. For three days I bled, and the new condition of internal haemorrhage demanded another operation—an emergency to staunch the flow of blood and save the life which was fast leaving my young and helpless body.

When I regained consciousness some hours later, the surgeon was standing at my bedside. I distinctly heard one of his colleagues say, "What did you do, Dickie?" His answer, though dim and distant at the time, still lives in my mind. "I plugged it," he replied. One often hears the words "operation successful", because the patient is still alive when it is all over, but it must be borne in mind that however skilful the surgeon, no operation can be successful until the body has accepted the new conditions and adjusted itself accordingly. After convalescence I returned to Rhodesia. Within a few months I was going through exactly the same pattern of renal colic I had suffered in the past. The wounds of the incision had healed, but the cause of the trouble—the formation of stones in the kidneys and ureters—was still there. No doubt they came about through a combination of badly "kinked" ureters —which was clearly shown on the x-ray plates, and cavities in the kidneys caused by the bilharzia bug. Fortunately my extraordinary vitality enabled me to carry on my normal pattern of living, which included tennis, rugger, athletics, and, of course, my daily work. I just had to accept the renal colic attacks as part of my life. Exactly a year later I was put on to the train to Cape Town in a very bad condition.

After three days and four nights of gruelling journey—over two thousand miles—I arrived at my destination. Within a few hours I was in the hands of a very famous urological surgeon, who immediately started another series of x-rays and pyelograms (tests which necessitate the insertion of catheters through the bladder and ureters, until they reach the kidneys). Dyes were then injected so that the stain would outline the kidney's internal condition on the x-ray plates. I was then given large quantities of water to drink, enabling the functioning power of each kidney to be measured in relation to liquids consumed.

The following morning the surgeon sat on my bed in the nursing home and spoke in a friendly but rather grave tone. I was fascinated by his imposing personality, his good, strong and yet delicate hands, and his obvious intelligence. I was, of course, too young and to naïve to anticipate just what was coming, but when he told me that he was going to remove my right kidney in four days' time, I accepted the verdict as a matter of course—such was the confidence he inspired. That was in 1929. In similar circumstancs today, with my current knowledge of the human body, and the acknowledged power of the grape chemicals to dissolve stones and other foreign matter, I would have treated myself successfully.

However, several hours after the surgeon had left my bedside, there was a dramatic change in my condition. My temperature shot up to 104°. My pulse was galloping. My face and eyes began to swell and were as yellow as a golden sovereign. Everything was building up in true fashion for an emergency operation. My little drama was reaching its crisis!

Within half an hour an anaesthetist had taken complete control of my consciousness—and my life!

It was not until the following morning that consciousness eased its way—very gently—against the strange and distant bleat of the fishmonger's horn as he joggled down the street in his old-fashioned horse-drawn cart.

A few days later the surgeon again sat on my bed. This time he told me that he had removed the right kidney. He explained that I had been too ill for him to cut deep enough to remove the entire ureter. Consequently he had to leave about three inches of the tube at the bladder end, *with a small stone in it!*

He warned me that the remaining kidney might not keep me alive for more than six months and that the stone would probably cause trouble in the form of an abscess! What a bleak outlook for a young man of twenty-six, who believed that once the operation had been performed, all would be well in the future.

Thank goodness the spirit of youth is unquenchable!

Within three weeks I was lazing in the glorious sea, and

sun-bathing on one of the most beautiful beaches in the world, and my life took on a normal pattern once again.

I remained in Cape Town for about a year with gradual improving health. With the poisoned kidney gone, the system had rid itself of the remaining toxins. As the severe renal colic attacks had not returned, I looked forward to a normal and healthy future. This was not to be !

A high pressure pain began to develop around the area of the remaining kidney. As it became progressively worse in the months that followed, I began to lose heart. I became morbid and miserable. Then came the turning point in my destiny. I suppose that it was quite natural for me to believe that the vast medical resources across the oceans would save me from further trouble, and perhaps an early death.

In May 1929 *I sailed for England.*

CHAPTER THREE

LONDON

When I reached London it was the first time and I realised how insignificant I was in such a large city, where destiny was spreading its wings and beating thought into a colourful pattern. Here was power and planning, and in spite of the ugly economic depression then enveloping the land, and myself for that matter, my young manhood saw a vivid close-up of reality. A brand new world created a fresh desire for living; a new hope in the search for body-balance, and a new challenge to pain and morbid frustration which was fast overtaking me, and distantly calling for death!

I walked boldly into this new world in spite of my insignificance. It was a strange and sunless land whose incomparable beauty was far removed from Piccadilly Circus, the hub of the universe, they told me. My spirits were high as I made my first call on the famous Sir Arbuthnot Lane. He backed the theory of one of his previous house surgeons that a badly kinked ureter could be severed at the bladder end, and in a shortened state, linked up with the small intestine. It seemed that the surgeon, then in Scotland, was anxious to find a suitable case on which to prove his theory. My buoyant spirits showed immediate co-operation, but I must have been very, very naïve to have agreed to such an operation, which, of course, I did, believing it would be an end to my problem. Had it taken place, there would have been a different kind of ending—a very permanent one!

Sir Arbuthnot wrote a letter to the surgeon concerned, asking him to get in touch with me. I posted it just outside the consulting rooms in Cavendish Square—but no answer ever came! Did a Guardian Angel come to my aid?

The Senior Urological Surgeon in the largest hospital in south-east London became interested in my case. A new set of x-rays and pyelograms showed the interior of the kidney to be in moderately good condition, although the ureter was very badly kinked from top to bottom. This tallied with x-ray films I had brought from South Africa.

The specialist's line of action was to dilate the ureter in a series of cystocospies. These minor operations, carried out with an injection of cocaine, meant inserting catheters through the bladder and the ureter, to the mouth of the kidney, for the purpose of "stretching" the kinked parts of the ureter, and breaking down the acid accumulation in the narrowed sections. Unfortunately this treatment gave no material benefit, and the kidney attacks I was then suffering became more frequent and increasingly painful. The operations in themselves were sore and very unpleasant, leaving a negative and destructive psychological reaction. After the twentieth, I realised that I would have to face the truth—the fact that the surgeon was only experimenting *in the hope of giving relief*, and, remotely, a cure.

I was grateful for all that had been done, appreciating the personal interest shown by the surgeon, but I was compelled to change my whole attitude and cease my visits to the hospital; mainly because continued failure to give me relief and a possible cure was again breeding doubt and mistrust within me, causing my naïvete to wear thin, and my mind to forge a toughened rapier. I reasoned that the bilharzia bug had done irreparable damage and the sooner I got down to leading a normal life, the better.

With a natural aptitude for expressing myself through photography—and a certain amount of experience—I opened a portrait studio in the West End of London. When the kidney attacks came I treated the condition with draughts of gin in large glasses of water—hoping to flush out acid accumulations and impurities from the kidney. That, of course, was the easy way out—the line of least resistance which proved to be the cause of yet another problem. My professional career progressed very rapidly. Soon I was elected a Fellow of the Institute of British Photographers and an Associate of the Royal Photographic Society—but alas, my draughts of gin had developed into a habit of drinking. Adding insult to injury, a duodenal ulcer appeared, and in spite of constant medical treatment, it was to remain with me, on and off, for twenty-five years! This malady, incidentally, can now be treated by the grape diet, coupled with the right mental attitude.

It is always very simple after an event to recognise how a vicious circle of destruction completes itself, and to realise how very stupid it is to allow one's natural fighting spirit to be replaced by the stuff in a bottle, but, at the time, I knew no other way. I was now confronted with the problem of the ulcer as well as the kidney attacks. Breathing became difficult as the pain in the kidney area worsened, but I realised that I could not expect any help from medical sources.

There are many methods of healing, but the most popular, of course, is orthodox medical treatment, which, obviously, was not the best for me—and so I began to look elsewhere for help.

I now know that the body in itself is the greatest healer of all—if the mind is conditioned to give it a proper chance to do its work. In actual fact, it is the only healer! There is a tragic conception in the minds of most people that one has only to go to a doctor when something is wrong, and that after an examination and some medicine they will be well again.

I state now, quite categorically, that it is quite impossible for a doctor, or any other person for that matter, to actually heal, for the simple reason that the body alone does its own healing.

The most that a doctor can do is to assist that healing by ordering rest, the right types of food, and sometimes a medicine which will help rather than hinder the process. His most important task is to put the patient's mind at rest, freeing it from inherent fear. A doctor will set a broken limb but it is left to the body to do the actual healing.

A surgeon will operate and keep a patient in the theatre for as many as eight hours—sometimes much longer. He will, with great skill and absolute dedication remove certain organs, repair others, and when his work is done, he will say a little prayer; a hope that the body will now do its own healing after the necessary major assault upon it. *And the body does just that.* There is a complete process of re-orientation, over which the doctor has no control at all. Operations produce mental and physical shock, breaking down the natural rhythm and creating subconscious fear. Blood vessels are severed, fluid channels short-circuited and organs removed, *but one thing is absolutely certain.* The body will, of its own accord, re-adjust itself, and under the new conditions come back into its own cycle of rhythm, *unless the doctor has failed in his psychological approach to educate the patient to this undeniable truth, in which case another hypochondriac is born!*

During the past thirty years, nature's method of healing—under the care of trained professional naturopaths—has become more and more successful, and within the next twenty, must become a very serious challenge to orthodox medical practice, unless doctors show wisdom and courage to break away from their hidebound organisation of authority, compromising in the fight against illness and disease. Naturally, surgery by skilled and dedicated men and women will always be needed, but the call for it will be considerably reduced by the intelligent union of natural and scientific methods of healing.

With the passing of time, and my pattern of hard living, my condition gradually became worse, until a year before the second world war, when I became a patient in the famous *Kurhaus Hoven,* a clinic in the Black Forest of Germany, under the care of Professor Martin—a Nature Cure specialist who was reputed to be one of the leading diagnosticians in Europe. He showed tremendous interest in my case and my hopes again ran high when I discovered that most of the patients were either millionaires or world-famous people. Professor Martin was quick to tell me that after my right kidney had been removed, the other had, of necessity, grown to almost twice its normal size. I was also told that I had a peptic stomach which caused an over-inflated intestine to press against the pelvis of the kidney, causing irritation, strangulation and pain.

On arrival at the Clinic the pressure was at a new high; the pain almost unbearable, and breathing extremely difficult. Immediate treatment of colonic irrigation was prescribed; a complete wash-out of the large intestine with gallons of warm water and a minimum token of antiseptic.

The effect was spontaneous in its magical relief! All pain and pressure disappeared. *I felt normal again and this was a wonderful feeling.* The treatment was repeated once a week during my stay of a month. The duodenal ulcer was treated with a special diet and medicine; but within a few weeks of returning to London it was as bad as ever! Ulcers are usually caused by hyper-tension, with a resultant excessive flow of hydrochloric acid, and made worse by unmasticated foodstuffs passing through the narrow neck of the duodenum. Today these ulcers can be kept under control, and even cured without medicine. Treatment must start with a habit-pattern in the mind after the spirit has been awakened and elevated, when all forms of emotionalism, particularly that of anger, will fall away and be replaced by tranquillity. Spiritual influence, which is always pure and incorruptible, is like a magic wand working miracles on the mind and carrying it through to the body. All foodstuffs must be thoroughly masticated. Rest, as much rest as possible, is essential. During an attack, hot water sipped as often as possible will give instant relief. After several weeks of this treatment the ulcer will have healed on its own accord. *The grape treatment, however, is a guaranteed cure within three to four weeks.*

Back in London from Germany I discovered that without colonic irrigation the kidney condition deteriorated. My doctor in London—a very close friend—recommended a visit to Mr. J. E. R. McDonagh (now retired), the then world-famous Wimpole Street medical specialist, whose treatment was to get down to the very nature of the disease and its origin and prescribe a healing regimen, which, oddly enough, included colonic irrigation. It would have been impossible to meet a more conscientious and thorough medical man. His whole life was devoted to the study and research of disease. He had written many text-books and his ideas were revolutionary. *Once more my hopes ran high.*

At the Wimpole Street clinic I was given a course of twelve colonic irrigations over a period of six weeks. The treatment was punctuated by a series of spinal manipulations and general body massage. Finally, I was injected with a vaccine made from my own faeces before the treatment commenced. I was then warned never to smoke or drink again, as the condition which brought me to the clinic was diagnosed as *intestinal toxaemia*—aggravated by smoking and drinking alcohol.

I have discovered that these two habits, indulged in absolute moderation, are quite harmless to a healthy person with two kidneys and a sound constitution, but for people like myself and others with delicate interiors, they must be avoided forever, since the body manufactures its own nicotine and alcohol to the extent only of its natural requirements.

The body demands that all toxins, waste, dead or diseased tissues and other foreign matter must be eliminated within the cycle of twenty-four hours, through the four established media —the urine; faeces; perspiration and breathing, otherwise there is accumulation within the body, and this is one of the major causes of illness.

If everyone would recognise this indisputable fact and re-adjust their habits accordingly, illness in the world would be considerably diminished, and there would be little or no frustration, the end product of diseased bodies and minds.

The vast majority of Europeans live in fear and ignorance of themselves, and their real purpose in life. For instance, a headache—the spontaneous and automatic signal from an intricate, mystical and very wonderfully designed system—that the bloodstream is over-burdened with poison and requires immediate dilution with pure water, *gets the very opposite treatment!* Instead of water it is given various forms of aspirin which, in themselves are toxic ! ! The headache is relieved all right through the chemical reaction, but the cause is still there, and the poison of the pill is added to that already accumulated in the body. This, in time, causes grave illness. Anyone can prove this. When next you get a headache, drink as much hot water as you possibly can. The pain will disappear within ten minutes or so, and the toxins—the cause—will have been diluted and washed out of the body through the usual channels. This cure never fails, unless there is a mechanical obstruction such as brain pressure or other unusual symptom.

The alcoholic has another drink first thing in the morning and dies of alcoholic poisoning, as did two famous young people whom I knew quite well—Robert Newton the actor, and Dylan Thomas the poet. Had they trained themselves to absorb large draughts of water and lemon juice last thing at night, and first thing in the morning, to neutralise the over-acidised and poisoned blodstream, they would have been alive today. This simple treatment also breaks down the incessant craving for drink and helps to establish rational habits.

The body is designed to be a perfectly balanced organ with automatic digestion. Those who are fortunate enough to have been born with excellent health and sound constitution, should develop the wit to preserve them, through a rigid, self-imposed discipline, to offset the strains and stresses of modern-day living standards. Moderacy, rest, fresh wholesome foods, regular exercise and plenty of fresh air, are some of the ingredients to maintain wholeness, but the principal NEED IS FOR A WHOLESOME, ANGER-FREE MIND WHICH IS CONTROLLED BY A SPIRIT CONSTANTLY IN COMMUNION WITH GOD THROUGH THE PASSAGE OF SIMPLE PRAYER. THIS IS THE BIRTHRIGHT OF EVERY HUMAN BEING ON EARTH!

The object of this book is to pass on to others the positive and constructive knowledge I have gained through bitter experience, so that they may avoid the gradual poisoning of their bodies and minds through toxic foodstuffs and negative thought, in what we call a civilised society. The "uncivilised" cannot afford the poison luxury!

Mr. McDonagh's treatment was highly successful. It removed all the accumulated toxins from my system, and gave me the chance to start a completely new life, with a bright and happy future.

Had I introduced a pattern of strict discipline into my life at that time, as suggested by him, this would have come about. As it was, there were to be many more years of pain and frustration ahead.

I was moderately fit for about a year, and then, through absolute weakness of character at the time, I gradually slipped back into my old pattern of dissipation—burning the candle at both ends! I used the excuse that this type of life was one of the hazards of my occupation, which, of course, was utter nonsense! How very easy it is to be wise after the event!

CHAPTER FOUR

THE LIVER

Until eight years ago—after my complete and permanent cure through the remarkable healing powers of the chemicals in the grape, and, of course, a self-imposed plan of unwavering discipline in my way of life, I was still incapable of seeing as far as the horizon! It was, therefore, in keeping with my make-up at the time to put off further treatment from Mr. McDonagh. I had let him down and my conscience troubled me. His interest and sincerity was more than fatherly. I had felt honour-bound, after his painstaking treatment, to give up smoking and alcohol for all time, since I was unable to prune my indulgence to moderation. I was not an alcoholic as such, since I did not drink at all during the daytime—in spite of terrible hang-overs! This came in the evening after a hard day's work and a refreshing bath. I would meet friends in one of my many clubs or in the fashionable cocktail bars in the West End. I rarely went to bed before midnight—and then generally in a state of semi-consciousness. How utterly stupid and destructive!

The ghastly thing about social drinking is that the victims are quite unaware of the process of self-destruction which they have set into motion, and from which they can never fully recover. It only requires time to reveal itself in all its horror and ugliness. Moreover, there is a very thin line of distinction between these habits and those of the confirmed alcoholic, whose metabolism is ruined as a result of injury to the liver.

A simple method of toning that remarkable organ is to wash six to eight large raisins and place them in a small wineglass. Add the juice of half a fresh, ripe lemon—sufficient

*to cover the fruit and show a clearance of about a quarter of
an inch. Prepare before going to bed and place the glass on
your bedside table. When awake in the morning, stir the brew
and drink the juice, which will have become sweetened. Then
thoroughly chew the swollen raisins—and the pips if there
are any.* After several days you will become very conscious
of the tonic effect. The treatment should go on daily for about
a month, and then every now and again for short periods of
about a week, when the need arises. The therapeutic action
is largely on the chemistry of the liver—the body's most
incredible organ.

To be certain of knowledge of the functioning of the human
body, I attended a brief course on physiology at a South
African Medical School. I also studied the subject privately
in conjunction with the comparatively new psychomatics.

The liver, that dark-red, dome-shaped gland, thick-bodied
and very rich in blood, is about one-fortieth of the body's
entire weight. *It is the chemical laboratory of the body, and a
master chemist who never makes a mistake.* It lives just under
the cage of the lower ribs on the right-hand side, and is
anchored to the diaphragm. It moves with that muscle when
you breathe. It stores, supplies and converts foods. Among
other things it is a control point against that great enemy,
poison. The liver can lose most of its cells through disease, or
wear and tear, but as long as there are a few healthy ones
left, more and more new ones will be generated by them—
until the organ is whole again. It is quite a remarkable gland
which is not yet quite understood by science, but it has the
power to convert almost any type of food into whatever is
its need at the moment. It is the body's principal glucose sup-
plier, and can convert carbohydrates into this fuel, and, believe
it or not, it can actually make it from fats. When it has stored
its maximum of 20 per cent sugar, it can and does reconvert
the surplus back into fats for storage in different parts of the
body—the reason why overweight people should keep down

their sugar intake, and the foods which are quickly converted into this substance.

The liver requires "quality" rather than "quantity" for its healthy balance therefore a diet of simple ungarnished foods, such as fish, meat, eggs and vegetables, all lightly cooked, are the best for its daily needs. Most vegetables should be served uncooked in the form of salads, thus giving the liver ample supplies of chemicals in their natural state.

When general ignorance of biological make-up is overcome, people will demand natural foods, preferably uncanned and uncooked. This will be one of the methods through which universal illness can be overcome, since sickness is the end-product of a series of bad eating and drinking habits; errors which form themselves into a powerful and destructive vicious circle.

Listen to what Capt. Roberts, M.C., M.N.I.M.H., D.B-Th., says in his book, *The Encyclopaedia of Digestive Disorders* (Thorsons Publishers Ltd., London):

"Cirrhosis of the liver. This is almost invariably due to long continued and over-indulgence in alcoholic drinks. Although I have treated one case of cirrhosis in a life-long teetotaller, the possibility of non-alcoholic cirrhosis is so remote that it does not warrant special attention." The cure for cirrhosis, he adds, "is very simple. It is the completely negative one of avoiding even the smallest drop of alcoholic drink. Then, with the very plainest of food, and plenty of exercise in the open air, the patient can often cure himself without any medicine. Frequent drinks of dandelion coffee should be the only beverage; it will also act as a gentle, persistent tonic upon the liver, and will act as an excellent medicine, as well as a beverage in this disease." Capt. Roberts adds as a footnote that in all liver diseases and disorders it is important to avoid all fried foods, and reduce all fats and fatty foods to the absolute minimum. That ends the article, which is further evidence of the body's ability to heal itself, if given the opportunity.

I state quite categorically that every disease which is brought upon ourselves through bad habits, lack of exercise, improper breathing, excesses of food—particularly the wrong kind, nicotine tars, alcohol, and, believe it or not, certain brands of cold drinks, *can be completely cured by the simple process of rigid dieting over a given period, provided the patient has the courage, the will and the faith to carry out the regimen properly. I repeat that the body is a perfect healing mechanism which only requires fearless and intelligent co-operation from the mind.*

As I did not have the guts to go back to Mr. McDonagh, I visited a clinic in the country every three months, where, in addition to colonic irrigation, massage and special foods, I also had brine baths to remove poisons from the body through perspiration—one of the four natural methods of elimination. This kept me fairly fit for quite a while and enabled me to bluff my way into the army in the last war.

The brine bath is a treatment anyone can have at home, without either inconvenience or danger, unless there is a condition of heart disease. The result is both stimulating and effective in removing toxins. (See Chapter Ten for details.)

The treatment also has the effect of reducing unnecessary fats.

At this stage I was back in civilian life, having been invalided out of the army. I returned to my studio, and again, unfortunately, my smoking and drinking habits!

CHAPTER FIVE

I RETURN TO SOUTH AFRICA

After the war—at the end of 1945—I returned to South Africa. There I bought an export grape farm on the east side of a mountain in a very beautiful valley. The whole was flanked by a majestic range which skirted the Indian Ocean. Here indeed was beauty, peace and tranquillity. Away from the rat-race in London with its social obligations and negative repercussions, I decided that this was my unique opportunity to start life afresh with my wife and small child. Standing on the verandah of my home, *Sans Souci,* which overlooked a perimeter of sixty-feet tall blue gum trees—guardians of the vineyards from the devastating south-east winds—I felt a tremendous sense of freedom. It is difficult to find appropriate words to describe the awe-inspiring beauty which surrounded us; the silence and the tranquillity; the subtle copper-colouring of the mountains in the fast-fading sunsets and the incredible green blanket of the vineyards.

My health had improved a good deal. I had been drinking far less since my marriage a couple of years previously. Cigarettes were also down and the voyage had done me a tremendous lot of good. *Sans Souci* was about five miles from Somerset West, which had become something of an English settlement between the two wars—especially after the last one.

Some people, like myself, had bought small established farms on which to make a living; others were retired, and there were those who went into the city for business, but all were charming, friendly people.

There was a preponderance of Afrikaans folk in the area,

with their more rigid behaviour and moral values. It would be difficult to find more sincere, likeable, and hospitable people in any part of the world.

The post-war English settlers, however, were apt to be clannish, which is the natural habit of most people when putting down roots in a new country. With them they brought many of their national customs, making the most of their cocktail and dinner parties—no doubt to insulate themselves. For me this was utter devastation! Barely a night would go by without Eve and I being at one or another of these good people's homes—or they at ours. Resolutions are, alas, easy to make, but mine were soon broken. That is where I was so stupid! Like everyone else I was given the opportunity to choose from two patterns when putting down my own new roots, and weakly, but characteristically I chose the wrong one! This form of life was to go on for about six years with only a gradual deterioration of health. The duodenal ulcer was bad, and the stub of the ureter with the stone at the end "exploded" twice in the form of abscesses which responded well to penicillin and aureomycin.

Open-air life and hard work on the farm stemmed health deterioration and off-set the damage from too many parties. Then the mould of my destiny was again to reveal itself. Domestic upheaval was inevitable after seven years of marriage to a person like myself, and this, to my great sorrow, was followed by divorce. Eve was a serene person; very lovely and gentle, but far too sensitive to cope with my emotional outbursts. Decent people like her should refuse marriage with men whose drinking habits are irrational. The culprits would then take stock of themselves and probably change their outlook—before it became too late!

After getting rid of my farm I coursed my way to Salisbury in Rhodesia. I married again but not with any great success, in spite of Daphne being a very fine and beautiful person.

This was the beginning of another cycle, which, ultimately was to lead me to the discovery of the Grape Cure—the

*greatest and most certain healing media on earth—and the
dramatic and complete curing of my own body! This was to
take place several years later.*

After six months in Rhodesia my health took a very bad
turn for the worse. There was considerable deterioration,
principally, I think because of another domestic upheaval. A
prominent urological surgeon pronounced me seriously ill. It
appears that there was an infection in the bladder, caused by
an abscess in the stub of the ureter where the kidney had
been removed. He emphasised the need of an immediate
operation to prevent this unwanted legacy spreading throughout my body and particularly to my only kidney—with possibly fatal results! I had every confidence in the surgeon, but
a little voice within me said "No". I had hearkened to the
subconscious cry of rebellion against more operations—or
could it have been the voice of a Guardian Angel?

*The body has the power to re-adjust itself in every possible
circumstance, and surgery should only be used as a very last
resort in aiding it towards this end.*

Instead of having the operation I returned to London in
December 1954. There, another distinguished urological surgeon advised against surgery, and failed to discover any
infection at all!

Remorse at losing my two small children and the break-up
of my two marriages, had a very severe psychological effect
on my life and health, and so, in sheer desperation I plucked
up sufficient courage to see my old friend Mr. McDonagh in
Wimpole Street again. Treatment was similar to that in the
past and his advice just as sound and sincere. This kept me
going for another year, during which time I opened a new
studio in Beauchamp Place—and with it, the door to another
round of social drinking! By this time I was divorced from
Daphne.

*One never quite recovers from the subtle and devastating
effects of a broken marriage—the robber of the real roots of
life, and for me there was to be another malady—that of self-*

pity! It had never enveloped me before, but then, in my physical weakness and mental despair, I was easy prey. This condition was rich soil for further deterioration in my health pattern.

Man is not unlike a tree with invisible roots. He is difficult to transplant with any measure of success—once his spirit—the taproot of his growth—has been seriously disturbed. This is one of the main reasons for psychological illness, which points to the great necessity for all mateship to be established on solid foundations. I have never had need to visit a psychiatrist, but have wondered how they succeed at all in curing a patient. The real cure is to be found in love, with all its fearlessness and understanding; its beauty and grace. Love, with spiritual awareness, which is discovered and stimulated only through prayer. Tranquillisers are a very poor substitute, but these and sulphanilamide tablets were given to me when I visited London's largest West End hospital. I was in a bad way, but examination found no organic lesion in the oesophagus, although the stomach showed deformity with retention of secretion. There was also a coarsening of the mucous folds.

I was frustrated. I was grief-stricken. I was terribly sorry for myself and I was completely alone. For the first time in my life I was helpless and unable to take a grip of myself—to fight, as we are all given the power to fight against evil forces of destruction.

Again, in desperation, I took myself for the last time to see Mr. McDonagh. This is what he said in a letter to me the following day :

Dear Shackleton, All the examinations I made of you lead me to conclude that the trouble which brought you to see me is of the nature of a nephritis affecting the left kidney. The opinion is confirmed by both the blood picture and the blood count enclosed. Also by the examination of your urine which shows numerous pus cells, a few red corpuscles and some non-motile cocci, which, on cultivation,

prove to be streptococci. Once inflammation attacks a
kidney it cannot be rendered inactive directly. Hence
nothing is likely to be gained by advising you to take
internally, either a sulphanilamide or an anti-biotic preparation. Treatment should be aimed at rendering the cause
inactive. Holding the same to be intestinal toxaemia, which
you are aggravating by both smoking and over-drinking,
my advice to you is as follows: You should make up your
mind to become a non-smoker, and remain one for the rest
of your life. And it would be better if you could see your
way to drink no more alcohol. If the latter is impossible,
then you should take no more than a little wine, which you
should drink sitting down at your main meal of the day.
You should pay attention to your diet, and I am enclosing
some general dietary instructions to which you would
always do well to adhere. Whenever you feel you are
developing a kidney attack, you should live, while it lasts,
either on yoghourt or buttermilk. You should do your best
to have your bowels well opened at least twice a day, for
which you cannot do better than take one non-sugar coated
Calsalette wtih a tea or dessertspoonful of Normacol—the
two together before you go to bed. You should undergo in
my institution a course of colonic lavage and manipulative
treatment annually or every other year, for the next few
years at any rate. On looking through my clinic card, I see
that you completed your last course on 31st January, 1955,
so you can fix appointments at any time now to suit your
convenience, to undergo your next course.

During the course I will arrange to have administered a
series of injections of combined miasmine and an auto-
genous vaccine made from the particular streptococcus
which has been isolated from your urine. The prescription
enclosed is for some tablets, one of which you should take
after each of the three meals you have during the day,
which I feel sure will help to render inoperative the mental
factor which is acting so adversely in your case. If there is

any further information about your case you would like to have from me, please let me know; and in the meantime, with my continued best wishes,

Believe me, Yours sincerely, J. E. R. McDonagh (Signed).

That letter was written on the 13th June 1956. I began to feel much better after the treatment, and the health promoting spinal and general manipulative masage helped to revitalise me. The vaccine immunised my body against development of the disease.

Unfortunately my mental attitude did not change very much. I was still hopelessly distressed by the broken marriages and the loss of the children. I was without spiritual guidance and was being consumed by melancholy. *At that time I was that sort of a person!* I was too weak in body, purpose and spirit to withstand the impact of my depression with the fortitude so essential in cases like this. Consequently I was unable, and perhaps subconsciously reluctant to give up my excessive wine-drinking and smoking, which, I falsely believed would help me to forget. *Then, without warning, there came a very dramatic change in my condition. I suffered a great deal of pain and physical weakness began to overtake me. Movement —even that of simple walking—was* ALMOST IMPOSSIBLE WITHOUT SEVERE NAUSEA AND VOMITING. This put an end to my work and I permanently closed my studio. I now had to pay the price for my ignorance and disobedience, and I certainly deserved the punishment.

There is a very powerful law which governs all life. It is the law of reaction—the inevitable reaction! No act, whatever its nature—whether it be good or bad—wherever it may have been committed, can possibly go unrecognised by this truth—this bona fide *law of equalisation; this simple and natural law of balance!*

Recognise and assimilate this undeniable truth and eliminate a great deal of misery and unhappiness from your life.

In the unhappy state I then found myself, I took a final

grip and consulted Mr. Thomas Dummer, the then President
of the Naturopathic and Osteopathic Association of Great
Britain, whose method of diagnosis was radiesthesia (the basic
principle of water divining). He reported my vitality to be
very depleted. I was suffering, he said, from intestinal toxaemia
and emotional stress, superimposed on a history of renal
pathology. There were also indications of alimentary exhaustion; defective metabolism of foods, particularly of proteins
and fats. There was a very high reading for cancer toxins.
Although deep palpation of the descending colon failed to
reveal the presence of a tumour, he reported that the constant
localised pain, relieved only by sedatives, the progressive loss
of weight and increasing weakness, plus bio-physical data,
suggested a strong pre-cancer condition.

Thomas Dummer was a very successful Nature Cure specialist with clinics in both London and Paris, and many medical
men as his patients. He advised that I get another opinion,
and I saw Madam Maryla de Chrapowicki, D.Psy., N.D.,
M.R.I., who specialised in Haemato Biocrystallography. I had
met her a few years previously and knew of her fame as a
diagnostician of disease through the medium of the blood. She
found pronounced obstruction in the region of the splenic-
flexure and upper part of the descending colon, which could
be malignant, she said, but indications were not definite. The
whole endocrine system appeared to have been strongly over-
stimulated, particularly the pituitary and pineal glands. The
kidney, she reported, was working under high pressure to
compensate for the very disturbed acid-alkaline balance. The
liver was engorged and intense. The spleen was strongly
stimulated and showed inflammatory condition—the possible
cause of my trouble. The chemistry showed an excess of
sulphur in the system, producing a great deal of sulphuric
acid in the stomach and intestines, as well as renal calculi.
There was a deficiency of sodium and potassium. The whole
system was very dehydrated and the digestive system lacked
oil. Radionic reading showed very low vitality. These two

reports suggested the possibility of cancer, and I was pretty certain that an embryo had started. *Instead of depressing me, it created a very strong sense of challenge. We all possess this sense and when it is backed by spiritual awareness, there is nothing on earth we cannot defeat.* I discovered that I was quite unafraid of death. In fact, it would have been a welcome relief at that time. People who are desperately ill, with no hope of a cure, tend to lose the desire to live. My interest in cancer is tremendous, since I now honestly believe it to be curable through the grape treatment. Here is my theory on the origin of cancer:

First of all it is essential for you to appreciate the fact that the pattern of nature is governed by balance. A human being, not unlike a tree or any other plant, a bird or a beast, has its own particular equilibrium. The pattern varies in different people, but the essential roots of balance are always there. In mankind, three elements, or facets, group together in the formation of balance. The mind, the body and the spirit. When each facet is fully developed, as nature intended it— the body to the maximum power of its physical strength to expand without strain; the mind to the limit of its cultural mastery for intellectual progress in thought control and power to reason; and the spirit to the fullness of its absolute expression in its communion with God; then a person is whole, pure and in perfect balance!

In this balance he is invulnerable to disease! Nor can he fear or have doubts of any description whatsoever. Few people reach this state, but it is the unified pattern for which man was made and for which he should strive, individually and collectively throughout the world. *I contend that cancer starts its formation at the weakest spot in the body, particularly where irritation is prevalent, when the "balance" of the chemical system breaks down to a point beyond restoration, as a result of an accumulating over-load of toxins caused by physical excesses such as over-smoking; too much alcoholic intake; over-eating of the wrong types of food; too much* anger, worry and other forms of emotionalism such as sorrow and over-extended grief. Added to these causes there is also the spiritual unawareness.

I repeat that the body is a perfect, automatic self-healer and will always restore its own natural balance from day to day, since this is its natural and normal function. It is when more toxins are put into it than can be eliminated by the four natural sources within a twenty-four hour cycle that an accumulation of toxins takes place. It is then that a new pattern of metabolic balance must automatically be created to cope with its day-to-day functions, and, inevitably, this is exactly what happens. Unfortunately, this re-adjustment of metabolism is on an unnatural level with a great strain on all organs. At this stage it is on an emergency level! A new chemical pattern is thus born within a vicious circle! The metabolism is compelled to accept the over-load of toxins, until it, too, in its new state, also breaks down. Then another unnatural and compulsory re-adjustment is made, until the constant over-loading of poisons from day to day breaks it down as well. This pattern is indefinite over a period of years —until saturation point is reached—until the spirit can no longer cope with the lavish and impossible demands of the flesh—like the last straw which broke the camel's back! It is at this exact moment, however, that cell growth gets completely out of control at the weakest spot—where toxic accumulation is at its greatest, and forms itself into a malignant growth. I am also confident that this "over-all" state of imbalance in the blood can be inherited by a new-born child. I am told on very good authority that the average person over the age of sixty who is operated on has cancer in some form or another. I believe the proportion is about 70 per cent. This is easily understood if my theory is accepted, but there need not be cause for alarm. If the body is poisoned by a gradual process, to a point of absolute breakdown; the bloodstream can be purified by a gradual process until all glands are freed of their toxins, and this is exactly what the ordinary

*table grape's chemicals do to the blood, in its contribution
towards the defeat of disease.*

*The grape treatment is a regimented process of absolute
purification of the bloodstream, and the destruction and
removal of every diseased cell in the body, without harm or
loss of energy. Weight is lost to the extent of three to eight
pounds a week—sometimes more, without danger during the
three to four weeks duration of the treatment. As the chemicals in the grape dissolve the toxins and all other foreign
matter, little by little each day, and eject them through the
urine, the stools, the lungs through breathing and the skin
with perspiration, so does it synonomously heal the mind of all
its frustrations.*

If my theory on the cause of cancer is correct, all weak
and ignorant people who persist in putting more toxins into
the body than can be removed in the twenty-four hour cycle,
make themselves vulnerable to the disease. Equally, all people
who do the grape treatment must, by the same law, cleanse
thmselves of the disease if it has already started.

When a man is very ill, especially if he is sensitive, self-
discipline is almost impossible. Severe suffering and frustration
require the warmth, confidence and understanding of a good
woman, or the specialised care of a modern hospital. The
state of my health at that time could not have been worse
without instant death—and I was living completely alone in
my flat. This was disastrous, but however ill one may be,
there is always a ray of hope, and it does spring eternal! My
hope came with a flight of thought which sparked off a subconscious inspiration prompting me to return to South Africa
to do the grape treatment, about which I knew absolutely
nothing. Ten years earlier, when I bought *Sans Souci* from
Baron von Lieres, he casually mentioned that in Germany
there were many clinics successfully treating patients of all
diseases on nothing but grapes.

I booked a passage to return to South Africa within six
weeks—in January 1957, but actually left a month earlier,

because my condition was so serious. The voyage had the usual stimulating effect. On arrival in Cape Town a fortnight later, I set myself up in a small flat on the beach front in Sea Point, where treatment could be carried out under ideal conditions, with plenty of fresh air and opportunity for sunbathing and long walks on the beach.

The effects of severe illness can be terribly evil when it gets a grip, but loneliness can be infinitely worse. It is in itself an illness! The two combined are devastating! I was apprehensive of this terror, since I have been surrounded by friends all my life, and I was in great need of human understanding and moral encouragement for the experiment. Then a pungent thought took control. I became acutely aware of the fallibility and general insincerity of what we call friendship, and the danger of my experiment being wrecked for the want of proper understanding.

I then became vividly aware that there comes a time in our lives when we are compelled to face our own problems absolutely alone, looking deep into our conscience and the pattern of our lives; a time when no other living person can be of help; a poignant moment when we must reach beyond ourselves, into the Divine Pattern for strength and understanding. Instead of calling in friends, I did just that! And so I was comforted.

At that stage the kidney had almost ceased to function. The pain was more than I could bear, it seemed, and yet I endured it somehow. My mental outlook had improved considerably, since I had refuted the challenge of death and accepted the Divine Inspiration which had come upon me.

I was aware of the gravity of my condition but saw no point in sending for a doctor who would only have given me drugs—and this story would never have been written!

I have a tremendous respect and affection for those dedicated men and women in the medical profession who devote their lives to their calling, but I would be failing in courage and duty were I to neglect criticism of their excessive and indiscriminative use of antibiotics and other modern drugs, in place of natural methods of healing. I have seen so much irreparable damage done by drugs, *and everyone knows about the unfortunate little children born in different parts of the world, limbless and distorted, in the name of dividends for big business!*

Listen to what Professor Douw. G. Steyn (whom I talk about in Chapter Thirteen) regarded as one of the foremost toxicologists in the world, has to say about antibiotics:

Antibiotics are very extensively used in some countries in feed in order to promote growth in young animals. This is also permitted in the Republic of South Africa. The author is opposed to the use of antibiotics as food preservatives for the following reasons: (1) They are prone to increase the coagulability of the blood, thus aggravating the already very serious problem of thrombosis. (2) Their continual administration or ingestion, induces the development of pronounced resistance in pathogenic organisms which are naturally susceptible to them. In the treatment of diseases with antibiotics, acquired drug-resistance by the pathogenic organisms has become a major problem. Of almost equal importance is the problem of acquired hypersensitivity in the human being to this group of drugs. (3) If administered in repeated small quantities they suppress the growth of virulent pathogenic organisms, with the result that less virulent organisms, which are not susceptible to antibiotics, increase and cause disease and death. For example, patients undergoing treatment with antibiotics are rendered extremely susceptible to infections with pathogenic fungi (aspergillosis and moniliasis). (4) They not only suppress the growth of antibiotic-susceptible pathogenic organisms whose presence in small numbers in the human body is essential for the development of immunity, but also affects the flora, and possibly fauna, which are essential for the maintenance of health (e.g. members of the B Complex vitamin group preventing pallagra and ariboflavinosis).

Professor Steyn is very outspoken and it seems to me that patients who receive antibiotic treatment, *have yet to rely on the natural healing properties of the body to repair the damage caused by the drugs.* Any person who has had a full and powerful course of antibiotics must know just how devastating it can be.

It is quite impossible to interfere with the normal and natural functions of the body without disturbing the pattern of its chemistry, thus creating both mental and physical damage! Just when are people going to face up to the fact that they were created by God and not an international chemical laboratory! In another chapter I relate a personal experience to prove how drugs administered for an ear complaint nearly cost me my life and permanently robbed me of the greater part of my hearing in both ears.

In these circumstances I made up my mind not to call in a doctor, or even friends, and I did what I had done in London only a few weeks earlier. *I drank quantities of hot water, sipping it periodically throughout the day and night; with good results. The fluid diluted the toxics and helped to flush them out of my body.* I recommend this as an invaluable emergency treatment in any kind of trouble. Common sense alone tells us it is the right thing to do.

The grape season was due to start the following week. Since it was dangerous and almost impossible for me to assimilate ordinary food, I ate nothing but peaches until grapes were available.

On the 21st January, 1957, I commenced the grape treatment. I ate grapes and nothing but grapes for seven whole weeks. No other food passed my lips! Of course I also drank water. On the twenty-third day of the treatment, which was governed by the most rigid discipline, a miracle happened. I call it a miracle because it achieved what no human being on earth, medical or otherwise, could have accomplished. The very roots of an abscess in the kidney came away with all its blood, slime and sediment, and from that very moment I was virtually cured by natural means, where orthodox medical treatment had failed and surgery made impossible by the fact that I had only one kidney. This was no fluke. It was a perfect process of scientific elimination of all toxins in the body through its own mechanism. The chemicals in the ripe grape, perfectly balanced, are harmless solvents; dissolving all foreign matter in the body—even to stones in the kidneys without damage to healthy tissue. The chemicals are also eliminators in that they remove the toxic matter once it has been broken down. Constipation is almost impossible, unless there be a bowel obstruction. They are also antiseptics which disinfect wounds and cavities caused by the removal of accumulated toxic matter in the various glands. Above all, the chemicals in the grape are cell builders. During the treatment there is constant loss of weight—approximately four to six pounds a week, until the bloodstream has been purified— when all disease has been eliminated. Then, without taking any other type of food, weight becomes static for a few days and then begins to increase slightly.

CHAPTER SIX

THE TREATMENT

My first act before commencing the treatment was to weigh myself. Being just on six feet tall, I should have scaled about 165 lb., whereas 146 was registered on the dial. This included clothes and shoes. I then made a record of all my symptoms.

My eyes were very swollen and blurred. It was difficult to see clearly even with my glasses. Eyes always swell when the body is in a dangerously toxic condition. Neuritis was constant in my right arm. The kidney was very painful and reluctant to function normally. There was pain on the left side of the large intestines. My ears had an infection and were very itchy. The stub of the ureter on the right side—where the kidney had been removed nearly thirty years previously—was painful and under strain. I felt extremely nauseated—and I had been constipated for several days.

I must now remind readers that I knew absolutely nothing about the method and routine of the grape treatment—and I had no means of finding out. I relied on common sense which told me that unless a disease could be pin-pointed and successfully treated with drugs—the only alternative was to follow the pattern of nature—that used by the animals; the gradual removal of toxins by fasting. This I would have been compelled to do had Baron von Lieres not told me about cures through eating grapes.

I recalled that the human body was a natural healing agent itself, and my faith in this became strong and remained so throughout the treatment. I knew that the human body was almost indestructible—short of deliberate mutilation. I reasoned that as it had withstood the full impact of my constant abuse of it for years on end, it would readily respond in a positive manner to any form of natural assistance given during its own period of self-healing. A period, at least, when it would be given the opportunity to heal.

One more important factor strengthened my resolve for do-it-yourself treatment. *Medical opinion from the very highest authority had made it quite clear that once inflammation attacks a kidney it cannot be rendered inactive directly, and that Sulphanilamide and antibiotic preparations were useless. That was emphasized in Mr. McDonagh's letter to me on 13th June, 1956. This is also proved by the fact that diseased kidneys are removed from the body!*

In the circumstances death was almost certain unless some kind of miracle was to happen. With the grape treatment I was strong in my conviction that I stood a very good chance of recovery, since it was a method of removing small quantities of poison from the body each day, without putting any more into it, as is the case with drugs!

After weighing myself, I bought half a dozen pounds of ripe, sweet grapes. I chose two varieties and divided the bunches into small units of about six berries each. I placed the fruit in a gallon of hot water and agitated for better washing, changing the water three times, since I knew that ripening grapes, and nearly all fruit for that matter, were being sprayed with deadly poisonous insecticides such as Parathion, which are not always rendered harmless by the time the fruit is ready for eating. I then planned to eat grapes as and when I felt the desire to do so, at any time of the day or night, thoroughly masticating and swallowing the skins and as many of the pips as possible.

It is absolutely essential that the bowels be opened at least every two days, as the faeces and the urine are the main channels of toxic elimination. I reasoned correctly that the skins would supply the necessary "roughage" for the contracting muscles in the large intestine to work on, and that the pips might have some medical property. *If the bowels do not work regularly it is absolutely essential to take a warm enema, or a glycerin suppository, which is inserted in the rectum and is effective within ten minutes.*

THE GRAPE TREATMENT MEANS LIVING ON FRESH, WELL-WASHED, RIPE AND SWEET GRAPES FOR A LIMITED PERIOD TO BE DETERMINED BY ONE'S DAILY CONDITION AND THE NATURE OF THE ILLNESS. NO OTHER FOOD OF ANY DESCRIPTION MAY BE EATEN; NOR MUST THERE BE SMOKING OR DRINKING OF ANY LIQUIDS OTHER THAN BOILED WATER—PREFERABLY HOT WHEN FEELING SLIGHTLY NAUSEATED AND COLD WHEN MERELY THIRSTY. NEITHER MAY DRUGS OR APERIENTS BE TAKEN IN ANY CIRCUMSTANCES. UNLESS THESE CONDITIONS ARE SELF-IMPOSED, VOLUNTARILY, AND CARRIED OUT TO THE LETTER, IT IS A COMPLETE WASTE OF TIME TO ATTEMPT THE TREATMENT!

Loss of weight will vary from three to eight pounds per week, depending on one's storage of fats. It could be more but there must never be cause for alarm. The treatment is absolutely safe. The cure is actually brought about in a very simple manner.

I repeat, the chemicals in the grape are a perfect solvent, and the fruit must now be regarded for what it is—a medicine! They will dissolve all foreign matter in the body without harming healthy tissue. This is a guarantee! Secondly, the chemicals act as an eliminator. Provided that most of the skins and some of the pips are eaten, constipation is almost impossible—unless there is a blockage in the intestine through a tumour or other obstruction, in which case an enema or glycerin suppository should be used. Thirdly, the chemicals are an antiseptic. You may prove this quite easily. Dilute pure, fresh grape juice with 50 per cent spring or boiled water (otherwise it is too strong) and apply to any open wound. Cleansing and healing will be far quicker than most remedies. Therefore, as the grape chemicals destroy foreign matter in the body, and eliminate, they also heal any wound, such as a cavity from an abscess. Finally, the grape chemicals act as cell builders. As I have already pointed out, loss of weight during treatment is constant, but as soon as all poisons have been dissolved and eliminated from the system, weight becomes static for a few days and then begins to increase without any other food being eaten.

I have so often been asked just why the grape treatment is so miraculous in its healing—and not any other fruit.

There may be fruits which will heal equally well, but I do not know of any. I doubt whether there is one whose chemical composition can measure up to that of the grape as a blood-cleaner and aid to healing. *The grape chemicals have nutritive value and therapeutic action, which are essentially due to the compounds in the pulp; sugars, vitamins, organic acids, mineral salts and ferments.*

The nutritive power is due to the presence of sugars in the grape—a higher percentage than in any other fruit! These sugars—glucose and fructose—can be used by the organism without the aid of insulin. Due to the facility of assimilation, the compounds in the grape favour the renewal of tissues, giving renewed life and vitality to exhausted and debilitated organisms.

Since the sugars of the grape burn very rapidly, our organisms are given an extra amount of energy, thus saving proteins, which are so important to the biological economy of man.

No less important are the therapeutic properties of other components of the grape, which, as well as the sugar, also contain all the vitamins from A to C (A, B1, B2, PP and C), the importance of which is too well known to be emphasized any further.

Another wonderful feature of the grape is the presence of organic acids (Malic, Citric, Tartaric, etc.) which, though in small quantities as such, are in greater quantities as salts (Potassium, Sodium, Calcium, Phosphorus and Iron), conferring on the grape the power to combat a state of acidosis which can be produced in the organism by pathogenic causes, or simply through an excessive consumption of protein foods. These mineral salts, when dissolved in metabolic water —that is the water generated by the wonderful and magic powers of life—as well as contributing to the alkalizing effects, cause a diuretic action by no means inferior to the best natural mineral waters. They also, in synergic action with the vitamins, make the grape a real tonic for the organisms, especially for children.

Finally, we should not undervalue the utility of ferments for their beneficial influence on the regularity of digestive functions, and to the beauty and freshness of the skin.

The information about the grape which I have just quoted was sent to me in February 1965 by Dr. I. Rossi-Compostella, of Hawling Farm Ltd., P.O. Box 44, Umtali, Rhodesia. He very kindly translated it from an article by Sabato Visco, Director of the Italian National Institute on 26th September 1962.

Dr. Rossi-Compostella, a true patrician, has the largest wine and table-grape vineyards in Rhodesia. He has brought with him from his beloved Italy many fine traditions, and Rhodesia will be the better for them. To him and to Sabato Visco I am deeply indebted for the invaluable information, particularly because it answers the many questions put to me as to why the grape is the perfect aid to healing, more especially in cases of rheumatic ailments, for which it is a guaranteed cure within a matter of weeks.

From Signor Sabato Visco's analysis of the chemicals of the grape, we learn two very important things. The first is that they are so well balanced that they become a natural and perfect antidote to acidosis—one of the chief causes of rheumatic complaints. Acidosis is the result of metabolic imbalance, caused by eating the wrong combination of foods, cooked at times in the wrong utensils; as well as inharmonious thinking—the chief enemy being anger!

During my treatment I discovered that the grape is one of the purest foods one can eat—if not the purest, enabling the body gradually to purify and heal through its own automatic mechanism. So pure and perfectly balanced are the chemicals in the grape, that it is impossible for the fruit to go bad. This chemical reaction just cannot take place. Instead it dehydrates and becomes a raisin which will keep for unlimited periods. When the tough skin is punctured or ruptured where it meets the stalk it can ferment or become mildewed.

I actually started eating grapes on the afternoon of the first day, after taking two calsalettes the night before. *It is very necessary to start the treatment on an empty stomach with a clean intestine.* The result was good but the waste was strong with chemical odour. The pain on the left side of the bowels was considerably relieved after the movement, which indicated some sort of obstruction. I awakened at 5 a.m. the next morning and started eating grapes again. All morning I had a severe headache and a strong urge to vomit. I drank a pint of hot water to dilute toxins. I forced myself to take a walk barefooted on the beach, where the cold water, lapping the soft sands, helped to invigorate me a little. Deep breathing and sun-bathing—five minutes each on my back and front (which was increased by one minute every day) completed my programme. Returning to my flat I read, relaxed and then went to sleep feeling drowsy. Throughout the day, at odd intervals, I ate grapes, drinking hot water after each meal—after a lapse of about an hour. *Water must not be taken until at least an hour after eating the fruit, otherwise it dilutes the strength of the chemicals.*

I consumed four pounds of grapes during the first day.

On the second, all symptoms were much the same as the first, with the headache and nausea still rather bad. There was a great deal of belching. I repeated my beach routine, my relaxation and sleep, but in the afternoon I went to a cinema to combat perhaps the only drawback in the whole treatment—boredom! A very small price to pay for such magnificent results!

On the third day I bought grapes from an old Greek

gentleman and was richly rewarded with a strengthening of my faith and purpose in the treatment. Explaining my need for really ripe and sweet berries, he kindly permitted me to choose especially ripe bunches from his trays. Then, quite casually, he told me of a relation of his in Greece who was chair-ridden for forty years with chronic rheumatism and was completely cured by eating nothing but grapes and water-melon for a given period. *What a tremendous fillip this heartening news gave me!* On the third day there was a slight improvement in all symptoms, although my head ached rather badly—a clear sign I felt, of poisons being harassed and removed from the body, first through the bloodstream, causing irritation in the brain during normal circulation. Bowels worked well but were sour in odour. I made a point of always urinating in a clear glass receptacle so that colour and unusual matter could be observed. The odour was strong. I kept up my planned routine.

In the afternoon a feeling of moral strength mounted as I became conscious of a physical freshness for the first time in many years. On the fourth day I awakened at 5.30 a.m. All symptoms were greatly relieved but headache was still severe. After the usual routine I went to bed at 6.30 p.m., my usual time, feeling very tired but with no signs of actual weakness and certainly no desire for ordinary food.

You will observe that during the first four days the only symptom which became worse was the headache, and at this point I will explain the reason for this, particularly because during the past six years I have come across a great number of people who have given up the grape treatment through fear and ignorance of what is really taking place, because of the headaches during the first four days.

Under the title of *About the Grape Cure,* Thorsons Publishers in London published the story I am now re-writing in an abbreviated form in their "About" series, which was limited to 20,000 words; quite insufficient for me to give a really comprehensive explanation of the whole treatment.

In April 1964 the booklet went into a second edition, but at the beginning of 1965 I withdrew it from circulation in spite of the fact that the publishers wanted to print a third edition, *because I needed to explain more fully the details and reactions of the treatment, with a special emphasis on the headaches.*

In an earlier chapter I spoke about toxin-accumulation in the body; those which could not be eliminated within the twenty-four hour cycle permitted by the system. To understand the reason for the headaches, it is necessary to understand the toxin-accumulation pattern. The best analogy is the ordinary domestic kitchen kettle. Constant boiling of water leaves deposits which cling to the side of the vessel, which is called "furring". Unless this is removed daily with a chemical, the spout becomes narrowed and sometimes clogged. To remove the chemical deposit one applies acid—the most common being domestic vinegar. The principle of accumulation of toxic matter in the body is exactly similar, but instead of drinking vinegar which would over-acidise the system, *we eat the grape whose chemicals dissolve the poison deposits in every part of the body, carrying them through the blood-stream to the four departments of excretion. On the journey the blood has to travel to the brain. Its very toxic condition causes severe irritation, in other words a* HEADACHE! *There-fore these headaches should be welcomed for what they really are—positive evidence that the grape treatment is really doing its job thoroughly, and so, in no circumstances should the treatment be stopped. Nor should anything other than hot water be taken to ease the pain.*

During the treatment, headaches vary considerably in both intensity and activity, according to the amount of toxins in the body being disturbed. A very sick person would suffer as I did. A mild disease would mean less frequent attacks of a milder nature. Generally speaking they occur only during the first two days and then quite infrequently.

Where the toxic condition is severe they can go into the

fifth day. We must recognise these headaches as a barometer of our real condition. When a person, unused to alcohol, consumes too much at a party, he has a "hang-over" the following morning—a severe headache. He is actually suffering from a mild state of alcoholic poisoning, which he checks with a neutralising agent—usually some brand of aspirin, which, in itself, is a poison. Instead, large draughts of hot water are the best and safest method of restoring the acid-alkaline balance of the blood, with the addition of the juice of a lemon—nature's best alkaliser. Nothing in life can be static. Accumulated poisons in the body are active. They set up a destructive cycle of their own making, and this is called disease, which, if left unattended, becomes chronic and ultimately fatal. Therefore the grape treatment is one which everyone should partake of at least once a year for no less a period than two weeks. *This is a guarantee for the prevention of serious illness usually caused through toxin-accumulation.* Medical statistics show that more than half of all deaths can be traced to arterial disease; clogging of the arteries, similar to the "furring" of the kettle, causing high blood pressure, blood-clotting (which is the first stage of a stroke) and many other side effects. There are very few people in the world over the age of fifty who can be rated as really fit. We all have some "hidden" disease which cannot be traced by diagnosis, and which only reveals itself when the body can no longer tolerate its evil effects—and then it is usually too late for normal treatment and an operation becomes necessary.

All the disease in various parts of the body is picked up by the blood, and at times is permanently carried in the blood, which must, by necessity, pass through the brain complex, irritating and disturbing it. Thus a sick person is always vulnerable to influences of evil and destruction without actually knowing it. He can rarely give or discover happiness for himself. Those who over-smoke or drink too much alcohol —both virulent poisons—without periodically cleansing the blood—are examples of this. Their impatience, anger and intolerance are visible symptoms of unbalanced metabolisms and sick minds. Drugs can only have a worsening effect—for they too are poisons. Whereas a person with a pure bloodstream has perfect health with a balanced mental outlook, and, as a general rule, an "awakened" spirit—the only route to inspired cheerfulness and constant harmony with all people in all things. It is almost impossible for such a person to become involved in crime or evil.

Science must look to the bloodstream if they wish to lower the crime statistics and the rapid increase in mental illness.

My advice to all people who do not feel "on top of the world" is to do a four-week course of the grape treatment, and then follow it every year with one of about a fortnight's duration—or longer if necessary. *This does not only mean longer life, but a healthier and very much happier one.* The treatment is the most thoroughly cleansing in the whole world. There is none safer, better or more pleasant, and the radiant health which one enjoys afterwards is something which no money on earth can buy.

Man will see that the engine of his car is cleaned periodically; his home will be spotless, as well as the exterior of his person, but when it comes to his most vital need—the cleansing of the whole of his innards for the maintenance of good health—he shows a sad disinterest and complete inability to cope with the situation, mainly, I think, because he relies too much on the family doctor, whom he considers to be some sort of magician who can actually see inside the body! Other aches may also occur in different parts of the body, quite unexpectedly. It may be in the heart, the liver area, the kidneys or even the joints. *These must be acknowledged for what they actually are. They are signs that there is disease in that particular area, which is being attacked well and truly by the grape chemicals in conjunction with the natural powers in the blood to destroy foreign matter. The longer one is on the grape treatment, the purer is the blood.*

In that state it becomes the victorious enemy of all disease! Therefore, in no circumstances must the patient become apprehensive when there are aches and pains—since the over-all condition of the body is becoming healthier each day.

On the fifth day of treatment my bowels did not function until the afternoon. The result was hard, dry and sour. Urine was clear but strong, with small quantities of whitish flakes. Eyes were still swollen—always a positive sign of excessive poisons dominating the system. I made a special point of masticating and swallowing more pips than usual, feeling that they would act as a laxative. My hunch proved right as the bowels functioned well the following morning.

On the sixth day the eye-swelling was reduced. Urine clear with less odour. There was general muscle weakness with a disinclination to go out. I forced myself to keep up the high standard of my routine discipline. Weighing myself in the afternoon I discovered that I had lost three pounds in six days. This was to become the average loss each week. It must be remembered that I had very little surplus weight to lose. From the seventh to the seventeenth day I adhered to my disciplinary routine. I was eating between four and five pounds of grapes every day, and drinking approximately three pints of water. Bowel function was regular. Odour varied slightly as did my general symptoms from day to day. Some days I would be completely free from pain; on others there would be a slight recurrence in the kidney, *which I recognised as a sure sign that the chemicals were now attacking this organ. I was right! As each little pocket of poison in my body was being attacked by the grape-saturated blood, there would be a physical reaction of pain, nausea and lethargy; the reason why reactions of this nature must be hailed with joy for the good that was being done. I cannot stress this fact too much.*

The need for ordinary food never arose, and there were no signs of actual physical weakness. In fact energy increased daily—far greater than is possible on an ordinary diet, because of the spontaneous absorption of the sugars into the bloodstream. This is one of the outstanding features of the treatment. Once the system has been cleared of most of its offensive waste, energy is actually at a "high" hitherto unknown in any circumstances. I repeat, the only real hindrance is boredom which can be mastered by the average person, when they appreciate the value of the final reward.

From the eighteenth to the twenty-second day of treatment my general condition improved considerably, but in every specimen of urine there was an increasing quantity of small whitish flakes—evidence, no doubt of the dissolving powers of the grape. The kidney was becoming more and more sensitive. There was no severe pain or pressure—only a feeling of "sickness" inside it.

THEN CAME THE TWENTY-THIRD DAY—AND THE MIRACLE!
I awakened at 6.30 a.m. I was fresh, and everything appeared to be normal. The kidney felt sound and painless. The arm was free from trouble. There was no headache. Bowel movement was excellent and free from unpleasant odour. The urine, however, for the first time, was very cloudy and the flakes had increased. The previous day I had ceased drinking water. The volume of the urine had increased. At 8 a.m. I had my usual warm-to-hot bath. Just before this there was a strong burning sensation at the end of the penis during urination, with only a few drops appearing. This was most unusual! Then small pieces of discoloured skin—one a quarter of an inch long—brown in colour and not unlike a transparent pea-pod with black spots appeared in the urine.

AT 10 A.M. I HAD A VERY SEVERE ATTACK OF RENAL COLIC —SIMILAR TO THOSE EXPERIENCED AT THE VERY BEGINNING OF MY ILLNESS MANY YEARS BEFORE, WHEN SMALL STONES WERE MOVING OUT OF THE KIDNEY INTO THE URETER AND DOWN TO THE BLADDER.

Only those who have been the victims of renal colic—and of course the doctors—know what hell and frustration a patient has to contend with during these attacks—when searing pain from the interior of the kidney—running right through the ureter as far as the testicles, is constant for several hours. There was nothing I could do! *Understandably my mind edged towards the precipice of panic, but I took a grip of myself and kept my faith—and before I had time to think again,* THE MIRACLE HAPPENED!

Earlier on I had taken several draughts of hot water to dilute the acid condition which caused the burning in the penis, and now I wanted to urinate again. IT WAS LIKE PASSING PURE ACID! *The burning was severe. Then followed a flow of slime, blood, coarse dark sediment, and many flakes of what appeared to be blood-stained skin-substance. This sparked off another tendency to panic.* I WAS ALONE AND IN DESPERATE PAIN. I KNEW THAT I DARE NOT TAKE A SEDATIVE, AND WONDERED IF SOME INTERNAL DAMAGE HAD BEEN DONE. SHOULD I SEND FOR A DOCTOR? HOW WAS I TO ENDURE THIS UNBEARABLE AGONY? THEN, IN A FLASH, THE TRUTH WAS REVEALED TO ME. IT WAS NOW OBVIOUS THAT AN ABSCESS HAD COME AWAY BY ITS VERY ROOTS FROM THE KIDNEY—AND THAT ALL MY PROBLEMS WERE OVER!

That afternoon I took specimens of the urine with all its muck to a prominent pathologist in Cape Town who confirmed the abscess breakdown. In this man, whose name I find I cannot divulge because of medical etiquette, I discovered one of the nicest and kindest people in the entire medical profession. He was quick to understand my whole story; the purpose of the grape treatment and its magic consequences, but, he warned me, I was very ill indeed and should straight away go into a nursing home under his care. This was a tremendous problem to which I could not give a spontaneous answer. In my heart I did not want to refuse the appeal of a genuine, sincere and highly skilled man who knew what he was talking about—and yet, had I followed his advice, would this not have been tantamount to failure of the experiment as a whole? *Of course I was seriously ill! Was I not suffering from the after effects of the equivalent of a major operation that very morning?* It was clear to me right from the very beginning of the treatment that a very definite process of toxin-elimination was taking place, with daily improvement in my health, and, had not the regimen dissolved and eradicated an abscess and possibly a stone from the kidney, where no drug could successfully operate? Surely it was the most logical conclusion in the world to believe that the grape chemicals would heal the wound caused by the elimination of the abscess?

My thoughts then went back to the very beginning of my illness; to the life-long pattern of pain and frustration—the expense and inconvenience of it all, and, finally, to the absolute failure of drugs and medical treatment to cure me.

With normal care I was confident that no complications could possibly arise, and so, with deep gratitude I thanked this new-found friend for his interest and kindness, *but assured him that so confident was I in the absolute healing qualities of the grape in conjunction with the blood, that I would return home alone and continue with the treatment, even if it meant my death!* And I meant just that. If my experiment was to be of any value to myself and to fellow-sufferers in the world, it was essential that no outside help should be enlisted—particularly orthodox medicine. Therefore I returned to my flat and carried on.

Within one week—still on the diet without any complications—I was 100 *per cent fit. I looked and felt twenty years younger, and I was literally radiant with health. All forms of irritability and frustration—from which I had suffered for so many years—had completely disappeared. It was quite impossible for me, it seemed, to get angry!*

All negative symptoms recorded before the treatment had completely vanished. I was able to read a newspaper without glasses. So charged was I with bubbling energy that I had to play golf twice a week. *Moreover, I had no desire whatsoever either to smoke or drink alcohol, and this state has not changed since.*

The gradual breaking up of the abscess in the kidney, and its final uprooting on the twenty-third day of the treatment is concrete and positive evidence of the power of the grape chemicals to find affinity with the blood in dissolving all foreign matter without damage to healthy tissues. It also proves that the treatment is harmless, however ill one may be.

Just what are the advantages of the grape treatment over all others? The average person can treat the average complaint during a course of three to four weeks *without having to leave work,* unless the patient has to do very heavy manual labour.

It is perfectly harmless since at no time is the patient disobeying any of nature's laws.

The process of healing is gradual and thorough and does not strain the system.

The treatment does not require the services of a doctor, although I strongly believe that they should adopt it when unable to get permanently curative results for their patients in such cases as:—Rheumatism; Arthritis; Migraine; Sinusitis; Alcoholism; Acne; Duodenal ulcers; Mental instability; Gangrene; Leprosy and even Cancer, and others, such as kidney diseases and Leukaemia.

For any chronic illness the treatment should never be less than four full weeks, as I never regard the course as being absolutely complete unless it continues for at least this period. It is a grave mistake to curtail the time factor because the patient feels cured. All residual toxins must be cleared out of the system—and that does take time.

More important is the necessity of completely removing the cause of the illness. Let us presume it to be an abscess with living bacteria. The grape chemicals work very slowly in tune with nature's healing pattern. After a fortnight on the treatment the abscess could be almost dissolved, but the roots would be both toxic and active. If treatment was to stop at that stage, the abscess would grow again—in much the same manner as an ordinary plant whose roots are left in the earth.

Complete elimination of the whole abscess must take place before the regimen is ended.

It is true that I did the treatment under ideal conditions, but I have conclusively proved, year in and year out since, in my own case, and in those of hundreds who have sought my help, that the average person can do a month's course without staying away from work. If a patient finds this a bit difficult after the second or third week, for any reason at all, it is better to take time off than to give up.

It is well to remember that once the blooodstream has been thoroughly cleansed, all disease will have been removed from the body, and perfect health will be the pattern for the rest of life—provided there is no further abuse such as over-indulgence in destructive living-habits.

I have often been asked if the disease can recur after it has been cured by the grape treatment.

My answer is NO! EMPHATICALLY, NO! *I have not had any recurrence of my original kidney complaint, although four years ago I was attacked by arthritis, as a result of strain from work and a shock from bad news. As grapes were not in season I was compelled to seek medical help. I visited one doctor and two specialists without any success. The doctor gave me a course of drugs which relieved the pain, but when the course was finished it returned. A second course would have been dangerous.*

I stuck it out for six months until the grape season arrived and after a course of three weeks on the fruit I was completely and permanently cured. There has been no recurrence since.

One woman who appealed to me for advice was completely cured of rheumatism, but a year later complained that there were signs of its return. I asked if she was eating large quantities of meat. She confirmed that she was. After cutting this out for a time she became normal again.

We must realise that most of the illnesses we contract are as a result, not only of over-eating, but of eating the wrong types of foods; those without the vitamin-mineral-protein-carbohydrate balance.

Acidosis causes rheumatism and acidosis is mainly caused by an excessive intake of proteins—epecially red meats.

Once rheumatism or any other malady is cured by the grape treatment, it will not recur if reasonable precaution is taken with diet. In a later chapter I give some useful hints in this direction. A really healthy body is the most treasured possession on earth. We should all plan to build and maintain it in a radiant state. After a month on the grape treatment I was absolutely and permanently cured—and I was radiantly healthy. In spite of this I continued the treatment for a further three weeks in the false belief that the small stone in the dead end of the severed ureter would move into the bladder and rid me forever of the danger which could arise from the ever-forming abscesses. I have said that the grape chemicals will dissolve stones in the kidney and the ureter, but in this case I was asking the impossible since the stub of the ureter was a dead end—a cul-de-sac through which no blood passed. The extra three weeks of treatment did, however, prove that nothing was lost by extending the period, and that strength was not diminished. *During that extra three week* period I took one Vitamin E pill each day (the natural oil of the wheat germ and not the synthetic brand), which gave me added strength and a sense of well-being. This Vitamin E pill must not be taken during the first three to four weeks of treatment.

Just what is the secret of the grape as a cure to practically all, if not every known disease? The answer is very simple indeed! The body automatically rejects all toxins through the natural process of elimination, so that the blood may become and remain pure, in which state it is able to resist all disease. If the blood and the mind remained pure there could never again be illness, but, being what we are, and living in conditions of stress and strain in unnatural surroundings, *we become creatures of imbalance* through weak and undesirable habits in every facet of living, more particularly with our food, drink and nervous tensions. THIS BRINGS ABOUT IMBALANCE ONCE AGAIN IN THE BLOODSTREAM, permitting disease to enter, breed and thrive in the body.

THE GREAT HEALING SECRET OF THE CHEMICALS IN THE GRAPE IS THAT THEY ARE IN THEMSELVES PERFECTLY BALANCED (that is, of course, in a ripe grape), VERY STRONG INDEED AND ABLE TO DISSOLVE AND DESTROY ALL FOREIGN MATTER IN THE BODY WITHOUT HARMING A SINGLE HEALTHY TISSUE. Added to this magic is the indisputable fact that, at the same time, the body is asserting its own process of elimination of all toxins BECAUSE IT IS NOT ABSORBING FOOD WITH TOXINS, OR TOXINS ON THEIR OWN SUCH AS LIQUOR AND NICOTINE. *The two processes make the perfect cure.*

So pure and balanced are the chemicals in the grape, that it is *impossible for the fruit to go bad*. This chemical reaction just cannot take place. *Instead the grape dehydrates and becomes a raisin which preserves itself for unlimited periods.* This happens even if a bunch of grapes is put into the refrigerator without any protection whatsoever. In three to six months the grapes will have become raisins! Many people have seen what they have thought to be a bad grape, but on examination it will be discovered that the skin of the grape has been punctured and that either mildew or fermentation has set in. *I repeat, a whole grape, in perfect condition, cannot deteriorate or go bad!*

CHAPTER SEVEN

DRUGS AGAIN

A few days after my miraculous cure, I received the urine report from the pathologist. The analysis showed red and white blood cells in profusion; a number of epithelial cells and mucus strands, and a good growth of B. Coli and pseudo pyocyaneus, which was resistant to all antibiotics, with the exception of neomycin 3000—in tests outside the body.

A very important observation here is that although the B. Coli was resistant to all antibiotics but one, the grape treatment actually removed the entire infection from the kidney, and this is really quite remarkable—something medical research teams should notice. On 23rd July 1957— four months after the termination of the grape treatment— a final report was received on the current urine specimen. It showed occasional epithelial cells and white blood cells, and a moderate number of amorphous phosphates. No red cells or casts were seen—*and the culture was sterile. The cure was complete!*

Illness is now one of the great and most prosperous industries both in England and America—one has only to glance at the sale-figures of antibiotics and other drugs to confirm this—*because disease is not* tackled at the roots— the cause is never removed by doctors. My own cure was no fluke. It has been done again and again by thousands of patients with the right mental approach; that of common sense, fearlessness, courage and faith, as well as the intelligence to realise that the treatment is perfectly harmless—being merely a natural aid to the body's own healing powers.

Modern drugs have proved themselves to be of great

value in healing, but because they are toxic, and because germs immunise themselves against them—they also do a lot of unseen damage. *It is impossible for a doctor to gauge this latter destruction which is known as "side-effects", but it can be pretty considerable, as everyone knows.* Here is a brief story of how I very nearly lost my life two years after the healing of my kidney by the grape treatment—by the improper prescribing of drugs by a doctor in Cape Town.

I was unfortunate enough to contract a fungus ear infection. I visited an ear, nose and throat specialist in Cape Town, who treated the condition for a week with cortisone drops, and during the second week with an acid solution. The condition deteriorated. I then went to my own doctor who took a swab of the discharge; had a vaccine made from the culture which was re-introduced into my body in a series of a dozen intra-muscular injections. Within twenty-four hours severe itching (similar to that experienced in the ear) broke out at the back of my head; under the armpits and in the groin. The ear condition itself became very much worse and commenced to pour out its acid-searing toxins all over my face. Antibiotic treatment was then unsuccessfully administered—and so I went to yet another doctor! He, a personal friend, assured me that everyone else was using the wrong treatment—and that he would never allow such a small problem to defeat him!

His confident manner and nonchalant attitude induced me to allow him to take over. He started by syringing the ears and then applying antibiotics—which amazed me as I was looking for something new. This treatment went on for weeks until every known antibiotic was tried—unsuccessfully of course. The doctor became so frustrated with his failure that he actually resorted to common detergents to syringe the ears. The next move was to cease all treatment to the ears themselves and to put me on to oral doses of cortisone. *For three weeks the drug seemed to be mastering the infection—and then—like a bombshell—came the "side effects"!* A sudden and ghastly pain hit the kidney—as though it had been kicked by a mule—and it remained there for many weeks. With the pain came a complete breakdown of my health, with the kidney suffering from a dangerous infection. *I was so ill that I was put on the danger list!* So concerned was this friend that he actually took me into his own private house and had his wife nurse me in an improvised sick-room!

No grapes were available in South Africa at that time. I became frustrated again and feared that I would not recover. I knew that a sea voyage would help and so I sailed for England once more. Unfortunately I arrived in London in the middle of a severe heat-wave. Within three days my kidney had practically ceased to function and I was taken to one of London's largest hospitals. I was given a five-day course of antibiotics, followed by a daily dose of twelve tablets of Hexamine Mandelate (this old-fashioned antiseptic was prescribed for me nearly forty years previously).

After a month in hospital, fluid taken from the kidney under an anaesthetic proved to be free of infection, and I was allowed to leave. I recuperated for a month in Devonshire and then returned to Cape Town, when the infection—Staphylococcus—flared up once again. It had merely been rendered inactive in hospital! I saw a specialist who warned me that unless I took sulphanilamide drugs every day for at least a year, it was impossible for me to be alive at the end of that period. This specialist was a very dear and respected friend. I found it hard to tell him that I would prefer to die making my own efforts by natural methods, than be killed off by drugs!

It was October and the grape season did not start until January. To ease the situation I lived on raisins soaked in distilled water for forty-eight hours. I supplemented this diet with fruit and vegetable juices—and the only solid food I ate was the diced diet, masticated to a very fine paste before swallowing. I survived until starting the grape diet in February for a period of three weeks—and the diced diet for a further two. Pathological reports on the 4th and 17th May showed the urine to be free from infection—and all cultures were sterile!

Once again the grape treatment had rescued me. I have been free from kidney infection ever since—and that was over ten years ago.

A tremendous number of people have sought my advice, done the treatment and been cured.

Three years ago, here in Salisbury, a parent approached me on the wisdom of putting his son—aged about nineteen years—on the grape treatment, because doctors could do no more. He was fast producing protein in the urine and the kidneys would not respond to treatment. He was, in fact, getting progressively worse from day to day.

I made it clear that what the treatment had done for me, it could do for everyone. He agreed to try it out with his son and other friends who were interested. Ten people, including his wife and himself, met at his house one night, and I gave them a lecture on the merits of the cure. They all agreed to start the treatment in the morning. I made an appointment to meet them all a week later. All were suffering from one disease or another, such as acne, rheumatism; haemorrhoids; liver trouble; over-smoking, and of course, the boy with kidney trouble. The week's treatment had convinced everyone that it was positive, and definitely worthwhile. Everybody's condition had shown marked improvement. The young man with the liver complaint passed the most odd looking worms in the faeces on the 4th day, and chips of stone in the urine on the sixth. I arranged for everyone to meet a week later when I discovered further remarkable improvement. The boy with the kidney trouble was showing vast improvement. At the end of the third week everyone was actually cured, including a case of migraine, but the kidney case, although improved beyond recognition, was breaking down on the psychological issue. He had experienced one or two negative days when weakness overcame him and he did not go to work. I suggested to his father that the boy got a week's leave and finished the treatment at home, resting as much as possible. From my point of view he just had to go on with the treatment—however severe the consequences, I knew that if he didn't he would certainly die. The father also knew this, and in spite of the fact that it was he who approached me in the first place to help—he now wavered in his faith—as did the boy—and decided to discontinue further treatment. Because I was not a doctor I was powerless to persuade a change of attitude. The boy went back to his previous diet—which was selective—and continued medical treatment without any improvement. Six months later he was sent to a specialist in South Africa, where he remained for a further six months—and then died! I think this case proves the necessity for the orthodox medical profession to make a series of experiments with the grape treatment in the name of humanity! I appeal to them very strongly, with all my heart, to do so.

CHAPTER EIGHT

REVERSION TO NORMAL DIET

Common sense tells us that a reversion to a normal diet again must be gradual. Moreover, food must be selected for its freshness and nutritional value; it must have overall balance in chemical compositions, proteins etc. New habits must be made when eating. Food must be cooked in utensils which do not corrode (see Chapter eleven), and it must be eaten in a calm and pleasant atmosphere. Above all, everything you put into your mouth must be chewed to a fine paste, with the aid of saliva, before swallowing. Perfect digestion is essential to perfect health. For the first two days after the treatment all kinds of fresh fruit and fresh vegetable juices may be taken, and, of course, grapes. Tea, coffee and chocolate should be avoided if possible. Liquids should consist of herbal teas and coffee, honey with a little lemon juice and water, sour milk and yoghourt.

At this stage of eating there will be a tremendous craving for solid foods—but this craving must be resisted.

On the third day you may have chicken and fresh vegetable soup with a little well washed barley added. (In no circumstances must tinned or packaged soups be eaten.) Uncooked dried fruits which have been thoroughly washed and soaked in water for twenty-four hours are an excellent addition to your diet. Toast made from wholewheat or wholemeal bread with only a little butter or margarine is also good.

On the fourth day the diet may be supplemented with steamed or grilled fish; grilled chicken and fresh salads, and very small quantities of other meat proteins if desired, although it is a good policy to avoid red meats. I repeat that the success of future good health depends upon good habits, and thorough mastication is top of the list. This good habit is worth establishing for the rest of your life, and to achieve it, much patience is required.

The need of a new set of values—with a well-balanced thinking and eating pattern—is of paramount importance once you have been cured by the grape treatment. It is worth going out of your way to create this so that your new-found health will be permanent. Good habits are just as easy to make as bad ones. Remember that once you have done at least a month's treatment on the grape diet, your whole body will be absolutely pure, and your mind clear, fresh and alert. The senses of sight, hearing, smell, taste and touch will be better than they have ever been in your grown-up lifetime, and your pleasure from them will be incomparable. It is worth keeping it like that.

On the fifth day, provided you feed on small quantities at a time of really fresh and nourishing foods, masticating everything perfectly, there is no reason why you should not eat almost anything, but it would be wise never to smoke or drink alcohol again. After the grape treatment the system will not crave these poisons, even if you were an addict. You will have a rare opportunity of fashioning a new and worth-while life.

"Seek and ye shall find." This famous statement refers to all things on earth and to all people. We need never despair, no matter what happens to us. There is always a balancing factor, if we will only take the trouble to apply our thoughts intelligently and fearlessly.

After I had bought my farm in the Cape and before discovering the grape treatment, I made a number of experiments with raw foodstuffs to enable me to survive. The diced diet, given below, is my most successful discovery next to the grape diet. It is invaluable as a whole meal, lunch or dinner, though preferably the latter, about the fourth day after the grape treatment. It has remarkable healing and cleansing properties, and will, if eaten regularly as a main meal during the day, actually cure rheumatism and skin rashes, and it is a guaranteed cure for constipation. If the diced diet is eaten at least during five days of the week, it is impossible to be constipated, unless there is a structure in the intestines. The ingredients are well balanced, and the whole can be considered a perfect food.

Ingredients. Two ounces of well washed raisins (preferably large with pips).

One medium sized eating apple (crisp—preferably Granny Smith type).

One ripe and well washed tomato.

Two ounces sweet milk cheese (Gouda)

Two ounces dry-roasted monkey nuts (no oils, fats or salt).

The juice of half a fresh, ripe lemon.

The seventh ingredient is saliva!

Method of preparation. After washing the raisins several times in hot water, place them in a cup and allow to soak in really hot water for about ten minutes. Then squeeze the juice of the lemon into another cup and add the raisins after they have been drained of water. This may be left for twenty minutes to half an hour. The lemon juice should just cover the raisins. Wash the tomato, cut into small pieces and place in a bowl. Cut the cheese into small pieces and place in the bowl with tomato. Then throw the monkey nuts into the bowl, finally adding the raisins and lemon juice. Stir thoroughly and the food is ready for consumption. In fact it should be eaten within fifteen minutes of preparation otherwise it begins to lose its own vitality!

Now find yourself a comfortable chair and relax with a little reading matter and your feet up if necessary, because it takes at least half an hour to thoroughly masticate and swallow the food. Remember that saliva is a very important ingredient! If possible make the diced diet your evening meal —your dinner, and don't drink any liquids until two hours have elapsed after the meal. After a week of this food as your main meal of the day, you will feel completely revitalised, especially if you cut down on other foods and leave out meat altogether during that week. The various ingredients can be adjusted to suit individual tastes, but no other may be added or taken away. The sweetness of the diet is controlled by the time allowed for the raisins to soak in the lemon juice. The longer the "soak" the sweeter the juice.

Another excellent food, useful as a midday meal is to take two young *mealies* (in season) and boil for about five minutes and then shred the corn into a frying pan. Add a little butter or margarine and a very small quantity of pepper and salt. The younger the mealie the less need for salt and pepper. Allow the pan to get warm to hot and then add a finely cut onion which must be stirred into the corn. Let these two ingredients simmer for about five minutes (keeping the onions crisp and only partially cooked). At this stage add about two ounces of diced sweet milk cheese (Gouda type with red rind) and stir in, holding the pan above the hot-plate. Now add one good sized tomato which has been cut into small pieces, with a little salt and pepper added. Stir very well and then allow the contents of the pan to stand for two or three minutes with lid before serving, without any heat at all. The ingredients are sufficient for one person. Masticate well and you will find this to be a clean and refreshing meal, giving good energy.

Steak Tatare is probably one of the most energising foods one can possibly eat, and is positive evidence that uncooked foods, retaining their own vitality, give this very force to the human being in very large proportions. If taken as a dinner without any other food at all, and no liquids for at least two hours after the meal, the sense of well-being the following morning is almost unbelievable. Here are the ingredients :

Take half a pound of raw steak (preferably fillet if you can afford it) and have it minced and placed on a dinner plate. (Lesser quantity can be used according to appetite.) Add the yolk of a fresh egg to the meat and mix well after sprinkling salt and pepper to taste. Then squeeze the juice of a ripe lemon over the mixture. The whole should now be garnished with sliced gerkins; finely cut raw onion and any other desirable pickle. No vegetables are required. Eat slowly and masticate well.

The digestive system is quite miraculous, being the centre of research for many generations by skilled and spirited scientists, but like the rest of the body, its complete workings are still a mystery. A lot of knowledge has been gleaned, but because digestion is controlled by the subconscious mind, its reactions vary according to the mental status of a person. It has, however, been discovered that an acid medium is required for the digestion of proteins which takes place in the stomach (practically wholly). Starches require an alkaline medium for digestion. Digestion begins in the mouth with the aid of saliva. It is therefore essential to thoroughly chew all starches, and all food for that matter, to a fine paste before swallowing. Fats and oils are digested in the Intestines, leaving the proteins and starches to their own compartments. Sugars are digested quicker than any other foods in the stomach and are stored in the liver as glycogen—to be absorbed into the bloodstream when needed. Fats and starches, or fats and proteins may be eaten together without imbalance of digestion, but it is undesirable to eat proteins and starches together (meat and potatoes) because the meat will draw an acid medium and the potatoes an alkaline. The obvious conclusion is that the acids will acidise the alkaline solution and the alkaline will neutralise the acids, rendering both mediums ineffective. I believe that we would all get tremendous benefit by eating only one particular type of food at any one meal, whether it be a pound of steak; a plate of potatoes; or half a pound of cheese. It may sound dull, but the benefits would far outweigh the disadvantages, and it would be far easier to prepare. It is worth trying this for about a week as an experiment. Variety could be established by ringing the changes at different meals. For instance, fruit for breakfast; cheese for lunch and meat for dinner. There are many variations which could make eating both a pleasure and a benefit. Even people who regard themselves as being healthy will find an appreciable uplift in their general well-being if they improve their eating habits.

Beverages can either be harmful or beneficial.

Buttermilk is a wonderful remedial agent and should be drunk as fresh as possible. It attacks and dissolves foreign matter in blood vessels, keeping the veins and arteries supple and free from lime deposits. It tones the stomach and provides ingredients to make rich red and healthy blood. It should be taken on an empty stomach in the morning at least an hour before eating other foods, or last thing at night, several hours after last intake of food or liquids.

Sour milk is another excellent liquid food. The lactic acid and lactic acid bacillus destroy the bacteria which decomposes food. This is extremely important to remember. It is best taken without flavouring, but if the latter is necessary, a little loganberry juice, with a small quantity of the fruit added after being chilled in the fridge, will help. This makes a wonderful and palatable summer drink, used at any time of the day. To get the most benefit it is wiser to take a glassful first thing in the morning—at least an hour before other food, and at night before going to sleep—preferably several hours after other food has been eaten. Professor Metchnikov said that Bacillus Bulgaricus, (Yoghourt) with its culture, favoured longevity and counter-balanced the toxic effects of meat, yet Dr. Szekely (*Medicine of Tomorrow*—Daniel) visited the countries concerned and thoroughly investigated the matter. He states: "Professor Metchnikov took the bacillus every day with meat. At the age of fifty-five he had the appearance of a very old man, and he died fairly young, although he believed that Yoghourt gave Bulgarians the highest statistics in the world for longevity." Dr. Szekely visited Bulgaria and the following facts were established: He found the Bulgarians to be a strong and healthy race, and there were more strong and healthy old people in Bulgaria than in any other European country except Russia. This seems to confirm Metchnikov's theory—*but he found other reasons for it*. First, the Bulgarians do not consume Yoghourt every day, *but they do take plain sour milk, and they do not take it with meat, but with cereals, potatoes, tomatoes and various vegetables*. They seldom eat meat at all, as they are mostly too poor to buy it. Being mostly of the Orthodox Greek faith, they have approximately one hundred fast days during the year, so that every third day is a fast day when they eat very little—a little fruit and vegetables and a glass of sour milk. Dr. Szekely found centenarians with black beards, black hair and perfect teeth. At the age of one hundred they worked on the mountains felling trees. Sour milk is both refreshing and cleansing.

Lemon, orange and grape fruit juices are invaluable, if made from fresh fruit. The orange has more vitamin "A" than the others, but less vitamin "C", of which the lemon is the richest. Grape fruit juice, mixed with a little olive oil, is a very good lubricant for the kidneys and urinary tracts, and if taken regularly will help to eliminate kidney stones. Lemon juice is lethal to the Diphtheria bacilli and to B.Coli. There is evidence of a bad case of urinary infection being quickly healed by three glasses of lemon juice daily—ordinary diet being given simultaneously—after all other forms of general treatment had failed. (Quote from *Foods for Health and Healing* by Dr. Dudley D'Auvergne Wright, F.R.C.S., M.R.C.S., L.R.C.P.)

Barley water. Barley is the least acid forming of the cereal family and is rich in carbohydrates, potassium, magnesium, sodium and calcium. It is, however, low in proteins.

Boil half a cup of well-washed pearl barley in about half a gallon of water. Let it simmer until the grain is swollen and soft. Strain off the liquid and allow to cool. Add lemon juice and honey to sweeten. This is an excellent drink taken hot in winter and chilled in summer. It has a very soothing effect on the kidneys.

Barley water, grape juice and honey. This is another fine drink which I have discovered. Make approximatly three quarters of a gallon of barley water (as above). Strain off liquid and when cool add half a pound of honey (a pound if you can afford it) and twelve ounces of bottled pure red grape juice (twice that quantity if you can afford it). I use that produced by Moni's in the Cape, South Africa and find it to be excellent. Store in frig and shake before drinking first thing in the morning instead of tea and coffee. It is refreshing, energising and cleansing to the system, particularly the kidneys. It should also be drunk at any time of the day as a thirst-quencher.

Pure grape juice in bottles can be a very good though not perfect substitute for the fresh grape. There are a number of firms throughout the world who bottle the pure juice of the grape in such a manner that preservatives do not seem necessary. During the past twelve months I have experimented with the red variety produced by Moni's Wineries in Paarl, Cape, South Africa. In conjunction with the diced diet, various types of rheumatism can be permanently cured. This also applies to arthritis, high blood pressure; liver complaints; bad skin, jaundice and many other maladies. The treatment is quite simple. The diced diet should be the only main meal of the day for the first week to ten days. Green and fresh salads and fresh fruits should be eaten liberally. Tea, coffee, alcohol and smoking should be avoided. The red variety of the bottled grape juice should be diluted with equal proportions of boiled but cold water, and drunk as often as possible throughout the day from a container kept in the refrigerator. It should be the first drink in the morning and the last at night on an empty stomach, at full strength. Before lunch a tablespoonful of honey may be added to the drink after being dissolved in a little hot water. This will have an immediate energising effect. I recommend sour milk for breakfast; fruit or fresh salads for lunch and the diced diet for dinner. After the first week to ten days fish and chicken may be added to the diet provided they are not fried. After another week or two the patient should be feeling on top of the world again, freed from all aches and pains and the nausea and tiredness which attends all types of illness, and at this stage can revert to a normal diet provided smoking is cut down to a minimum, if not given up altogether, and red meats should be avoided. In the cases of high blood pressure the patient should include well-washed raisins in the daily diet from commencement of treatment and continue with daily portions for many months.

Colds and influenza can be cured within twenty-four hours. As soon as there is the slightest sign of a cold or the first symptoms of 'flu, gargling with tincture of iodine must commence immediately. Put three or four drops of iodine into half a tumbler of warm water. Throw the head well back and gargle vigorously, and then allow the solution to remain at the back of the throat for as long as is bearable before clearing it from the mouth. *Gargling must be carried out at least three times a day;* first thing in the morning; just before lunch and the last thing at night, *and the treatment must continue* thus for at least five days, when gargling need only be done once a day. At the first sign of recurrence, gargling must start again, *because new germs are breeding daily and must be destroyed as they emerge.* The success of the treatment depends on all germs being instantly stamped out before they have a chance to set up a condition of inflammation. This treatment is a positive cure.

Diarrhoea or better known as "runny-tummy". This is generally caused through a mild poisoning and can be checked, as a general rule within twenty-four hours. The cure is simple though inconvenient. Large draughts of hot water must be sipped as often as possible throughout the day, and in no circumstances may food of any description be taken. The bottled grape juice may also be taken liberally. Once a day a tablespoonful of honey (diluted with a little warm water) may be added to the grape juice. This will give sufficient energy for the day. The patient should stay in bed and relax as much as possible. If the condition has not been cleared in the first twenty-four hours, repeat it the following day. Rarely does the body require two days, but in bad cases this may be necessary. When returning to food eat small quantities, avoiding fats and oils, and, of course milk. Dry toast with chicken soup and vegetables is excellent, if all fat has been removed. This same treatment is excellent for food-poisoning. I am rather prone to fish poisoning and only recently I had a very bad bout; waking in the middle of the night with violent vomiting and constant diarrhoea. The whole thing was quite uncontrollable *but I did not panic!* I knew that the only thing to be done was to drink as much hot water as possible, thereby diluting the poison in the system and removing it through the usual channels. By the morning I had the condition under control, after drinking two glasses of grape juice during the night. I spent a day in bed without any further diarrhoea or vomiting and the following day I was at work, looking rather ghastly, I was told, but quite able to tackle my day's work in the right spirit. As long as people don't panic they can see quite clearly what should be done. Since my permanent cure of the kidney complaint through the grape treatment, I have had the odd bit of trouble but other than for a hernia operation a year ago, I have always treated myself with hot water and been cured immediately, with one exception. I was spending a week's holiday at an hotel in the Eastern district of Rhodesia and got fish poisoning the second day. The manageress insisted on sending for a doctor because my condition looked bad. I consented only because I was a guest at the hotel. I was given a modern concoction to take several times a day, and the outcome was that I had to remain in bed for a week—with very little change in my condition until I got up. The medicine bill was preposterous, and, of course, the doctor's fees were high as he had to come from a distance. Doctors are so essential for very many reasons, but I do hope that the day will soon come when they will use natural treatments which have proved themselves time and again.

A year ago I went into hospital here in Salisbury in Rhodesia on a Monday afternoon. The following morning a very skilled surgeon operated on me for a bad hernia on the right side where the kidney had come out and where I was opened for appendicitis some years previously. After the operation I suffered a great deal of pain but refused any injections. I had brought three cases of grapes into the hospital and during the day I nibbled at them. The following morning I was feeling fine and actually stood up beside my bed. That evening I walked to the bathroom, as is the custom now employed in all hospitals a day or two after ordinary operations. I continued with the grapes for three days and then ate only vegetables and chicken. On the seventh day I left hospital carrying my suitcase and driving my car. I went to my office and remained there for two hours (it was a public holiday).

The following day I went to work again for three hours and did this until the end of the week. On the third day after coming out of hospital I kept an appointment with the surgeon to have the stitches removed. He asked me to come and see him in a week's time for a final check-up. Although I was working every day, the whole day, I completely forgot to see the surgeon and months later I wrote and apologised. The point is that my wound healed beautifully and quickly because my blood was purified through the grapes and my mind was completely unafraid all the time, allowing my body to do its own healing in its own good way. I am quite convinced that if surgeons were to insist on patients drinking bottled grape juice for several days before an operation—if fresh grapes are not in season—and grapes themselves if they are—and for several days in the hospital after the operation with only honey as an added food, not only would their patients heal twice as quickly, but the danger of complications through toxins would be greatly minimised.

Exercise and proper breathing is essential to good health. No human being can be healthy without a fair measure of natural exercise and proper breathing in places where the air is fresh. I have already said that after the grape treatment the body is fresh, alive, incredibly clean and highly sensitive. It is in the ideal condition to accept a completely new pattern for good living which will not only guarantee longer life, but certainly a very much happier one.

When you plan your new regime, remember that proper breathing is a most important factor. Every living cell must breathe because it needs oxygen to live, just as it expels carbon dioxide, the poisonous waste—to keep it in balance. It is mainly through breathing that we get oxygen into the blood-stream for distribution throughout the body. As we cannot live without oxygen, correct breathing becomes a most important function.

During one of the lectures I attended on physiology, I was very surprised to learn that the average person uses only one-third of his lung capacity throughout his lifetime. It stands to reason that the more we develop this organ, with an alert consciousness of its purpose, using a greater proportion for the intake of oxygen, *through deeper breathing*, the greater will be our vitality. It is the duty of every parent and every school to instil into the minds of their children the importance of correct breathing—and to see that they carry out a disciplinary plan to achieve it.

Hiccups can be cured in a few minutes if you take a paper bag and breathe into it. As you inhale so you will take back into the lungs the carbon dioxide you have just exhaled, instead of fresh oxygen. The automatic control of breathing is centred in the brain, according to the level of carbon dioxide in the lungs. When you breathe in this bad air instead of oxygen, the brain control centre calls for deeper inspirations which then regulates the contractions of the diaphragm, enabling it to break the spasm.

Earache. An excellent home-remedy for earache is to boil

two segments of garlic until soft and then add them to one ounce of pure olive oil after they have been slightly crushed. Allow them to stand in a small bottle which can be kept for a considerable time without deterioration. When the ear aches, shake the bottle and pour several drops of the oil into the ear. In nine cases out of ten there is almost instant relief, particularly if the oil is slightly warmed on a teaspoon. Continue with the treatment until the condition clears up.

CHAPTER NINE

HOW TO STOP SMOKING

Before I tell you of the value of the ice cure and the brine bath, I want to record a comparatively simple method to stop smoking. In effect it comprises four days of rigid discipline, during which time there is not only a substitute for the cigarette but a daily challenge to one's integrity. Probably for the first time in your life you will have the opportunity of proving whether you are a negative person with negative prospects ahead, or a real person with guts, with a sound will and the ability to put it into action whenever necessary, giving you a positive outlook for the future with assured success. Of this there is no doubt if you can prove that your whole personality has not been swamped by the insidious influence of one of the most virulent poisons known to science.

Smoking in absolute moderation is not in the least bit harmful. It is dangerous, and very dangerous indeed when a person is unable to control the number of cigarettes smoked during a day; especially when irritability dominates someone who is craving for a cigarette. I cannot stress too strongly the damage—secret damage—which is being done to the body through nicotine poisoning. *Every smoker who just must have a cigarette or become irritable is a positive case of self-imposed slavery of all the organs in the body, and a certain case of nicotine poisoning.* Once this happens there is daily deterioration of the whole system governing the entire body, until one particular organ has got to surrender under the pressure of its slavery. There is no doubt but that this is the beginning of cancer. Whether it be in the throat, the lungs, the liver or the stomach does not matter in the least. *What does matter is that the person is no longer human.* I have seen women sitting in buses and trains with a small child on their lap and a cigarette in the right hand with the smoke twirling up into the child's eyes. These women, most of them undoubtedly very good mothers and fine people, are quite oblivious to the fact that they are destroying the eye-sight of their own flesh and blood, and worse, that these little children are also developing toxic blood through inhalation of the smoke fumes. A non-smoker has only to go into a room where several people have been smoking and in a few moments becomes aware of eye and nostril irritation through toxic attack. The unfortunate smoker is anaesthetized mentally as well as physically and can never know of the damage being wrought. This is rather sad because men and women in high places must make decisions for the future welfare of their fellow-beings. If they are heavy smokers, and drinkers for that matter, none of the decisions made can be true, worthy and just. That is one of the dangers of the next world war. The people who will be responsible for the incredible devastation will not be conscious of the evil they are planning. Everyone must start an individual campaign of self-purification, in all aspects, otherwise they will be powerless in all things, particularly in any attempt to push back the fast moving tide of devastation which is flooding the world. It is only through a pure body and a pure mind that we are able to see truth and the immediate danger which always lies ahead—and do something practical to stem that tide!

For an addict to give up cigarettes always appears to be an impossible task because the will has been drugged to a point of absolute lethargy and uselessness in its major task of protecting the body. And this is a very sorry state of affairs which the addict mind just cannot perceive. It is also a very sorry state of affairs because nicotine poisoning robs the body of most of its vitality and the smoker is always looking for another excuse for tiredness, exhaustion and a colourless life which over-smoking always brings in its wake.

The method of beating the evil of over-smoking takes just four days. After that the intense craving ceases. What is left can be coped with quite easily. I think mine is the best-known method because it becomes a personal victory without any drugs—without any more toxins being added to an already over-poisoned bloodstream. It is a great personal achievement on which you will never go back. The system embodies quite a few psychological factors which should be studied. To get the best results it is essential to substitute a new habit for the one which is being taken away. The substitute in this course is a bag of raisins. Buy several pounds of assorted varieties, especially the largest with pips. Mix them in one large bag and take out sufficient for one day—about half a pound. Wash these thoroughly in several changes of hot water and dry with a clean cloth and place into a small plastic bag which you will carry on your person.

The first positive act in this four-day course is to throw away all the cigarettes in your possession at the very moment you make up your mind to stop smoking—and never leave your decision until tomorrow. Do it at this very minute! In no circumstances must you give your cigarettes to anyone. Surely it is not right to give to another person the very thing for which you have the greatest contempt? And contempt you must have for the cigarettes and your smoking of them, when you throw them in the dustbin or out of the window.

The next thing is to realise that you will never be smoking again in your lifetime, so that when a craving arrives for a cigarette, treat it also with the contempt it deserves, but at the same time chew a small quantity of raisins, which will check the craving and also have the effect of helping to remove the concentrated essence of nicotine from the lungs and the bloodstream. The third and very important feature is the drinking of as much water as is possible throughout the day, preferably hot, when the craving is desperate. This will remove the toxins as they are being moved and circulated throughout the body before being excreted through the four normal channels. Raisins should be eaten after every drink of water. Another very important psychological factor confronts you at the end of the first day, however great the craving to smoke again. You will realise that *you have actually succeeded in finishing one quarter of the course,* and that it is worth every possible effort of will to go on—and you will go on! At the beginning of the second day remember that you are going into the half-way stretch, and at the end of the third day it will be well to remember the significance of the moment. *You will actually have beaten the craving for all time!* Because at this stage it becomes less and less each hour. At this stage three-quarters of the course will have been completed, *and you will never be fool enough to have to go through those first three days again at any other time.* It would be madness, but it would also be madness to give up at this stage. If you will encourage your sense of values to appreciate these facts, which you will have created for yourself, by yourself, you will discover that the last day—the fourth day—will be comparatively easy to cope with.

I stated that the course will only take four days. In effect it must go on as long as there is the slightest suggestion of a craving to smoke. After the fourth day, however, the craving, the irresistible craving will have been mastered, provided all instructions for the course have been faithfully carried out. After a week most people will find that the craving has disappeared altogether, but I must give *a warning that under no circumstances must anyone succumb to the* temptation of having just one cigarette because they know that they will never again become an addict, since you now have control.

One cigarette will not bring back the craving, but it will have the extraordinary psychological effect of giving you a false confidence that you will be able to resist smoking at any time you choose. The desire to have a cigarette after you have mastered the craving to smoke is merely a habit-compulsion which should be treated with contempt and resisted with all your power of will.

Once you have completed the whole course, however short or long it may be, *never, never smoke again, whatever the circumstances.* You will then be able to look forward to a future which will be free from a great deal of frustration, backed with an ever-growing pattern of excellent and vibrant health.

The grape treatment will permanently stop people smoking, because from the very first day of the course the toxins in the bloodstream which create the craving to smoke are being gradually destroyed and removed from the body, but the four-day method is one which can be used when grapes are not in season.

CHAPTER TEN

THE BRINE BATH AND ICE CURE

As everyone knows, perspiring is one of the four natural methods of eliminating toxins from the body. The brine bath is an inexpensive treatment in the home for people who feel sluggish or liverish, and haven't the facilities to get on a horse every morning before breakfast. Combined with the ice cure it is invaluable in ferreting out hidden sources of illness in the body and curing them. This treatment may be used once a week, with great advantage.

Brine bath. Put from two to four pounds of ordinary coarse kitchen salt in your bath, which you can nearly fill with hot water—as hot as you can bear without discomfort. Agitate the water until the salt is thoroughly dissolved and evenly mixed and then get into the bath and relax. Every now and again turn on the hot water so that it runs slowly. Mix with the action of the arms and the feet. Stop the flow when the water feels hot enough but do not get out. In about half an hour you will commence to perspire freely from the brow and may feel a little nauseated with a rise in your own temperature. There is no cause for alarm, but at this stage a couple of glasses of cold water should be sipped and then you should get out of the bath and dry with a large coarse towel. The treatment is little different from that of an ordinary turkish bath but is very much more beneficial.

After drying you must get into bed, placing a large bath towel between your body and the lower sheet, and wrapping yourself well in another large bath towel. At this stage an ice compress must be placed on the solar plexus. (If you are alone this can be prepared before taking the bath, otherwise it should be prepared just as you are ready to emerge from the bath.)

The ice cure with compress was brought to my notice by my good friend the late Dr. Johanna Brandt. She believed very strongly indeed in the treatment and told me that most people believed that they were quite healthy until they tried the ice cure which has the knack of ferreting out hidden diseases and successfully treating them.

Take a damp turkish towel and fold it in half to make a square; then place six to ten cubes of ice from the frig in the centre, folding the four corners of the towel over one another as they cover the ice. The compress must then be placed over the solar plexus and the organs of excretion. The thickly folded part of the towel must remain on top to keep dry the bedding and the towel on which you are lying. The first water from the melting ice will be absorbed by the towel, and when the compress is wet and icy cold, the healing action will begin. There will not be any shock. A hot water bottle may be placed at your feet and then you must relax properly and go to sleep peacefully for two or three hours while the body is doing its own cleansing and self-healing.

If you are unhealthy and the bloodstream is not as free from impurities as you had imagined, the condition will manifest itself. There may be a fiery red on the flesh under the compress, or patches of discolouration may appear on other parts of the body, in which case you may be sure that there is internal congestion and inflammation.

Dr. Johanna Brandt says that if you get headaches, diarrhoea, heartburn, nausea, or a running cold after the treatment, or if you bring up bile or cough up phlegm, or experience anything unusual, there is no need to be alarmed. It is merely the evidence that all is not well with you, and it is only alarming if there was no remedy. The ice treatment will assist the body in removing the cause of the trouble in much the same manner as it produced the symptom. Nature always heals a chronic condition by first making it acute. Dr.

Johanna Brandt told me that the application of the ice pack to the centre of gravity, stimulates the blood to run to the frozen area to warm it, returning to the heart and lungs with its burden of impurities. The process should continue every three or four days for several weeks—on an empty stomach. The best time would be about five or six o'clock in the evening after work. If there are unusual symptoms the treatment should go on a little longer—as long as a couple of months and a strict diet should be adhered to, giving the body every opportunity, every bit of help, in its own process of healing. The special diet should consist of sour milk; fresh and well washed dried fruits; dates, grape juice and fresh salads with as little salt as possible, but with the addition of some cheese. The diced diet may also be eaten. An occasional glass of fresh lemon juice and water is excellent—one every two days. Vegetable (fresh) soup made with well washed pearl barley and a little chicken is a valuable addition to the diet. Honey should be taken once or twice a day as a spontaneous energiser. If you wish to have bread let it be wholemeal or wholewheat—preferably the latter—and have it toasted. After the treatment—the period will be determined by your own common sense—return gradually to a normal diet.

When you first start the treatment, you may feel that you have caught a cold through contact with the ice, but this is impossible if you have kept the rest of your body perfectly warm. One does not catch a cold after cold treatment; only heat has an unnatural, chilly and lowering reaction.

CHAPTER ELEVEN

THE VALUE OF HEALTHY FOODS

To maintain good health the best principle is to feed on small quantities of really fresh, nourishing foods, only partially cooked, and where possible not cooked at all, so that all the goodness is retained. Rather than write another book on dieting in general, I am sure it is wiser to tell you about books I have read and systems I have tried out happily and satisfactorily. The books I recommend are: *Dear Housewives* by Doris Grant; published by Faber and Faber Ltd., 24 Russell Square, London. This is really a wonderful book which everyone should read, more especially women with homes and families. The B.B.C. Woman's Hour comments:

"An excellent book . . . on the importance of using good, basic ingredients in our cooking. Mrs. Grant is deeply shocked by what she calls our lack of 'honest' foods—by the bleaching, dyeing, dehydrating, freezing and tinning, which makes a pretence of meat, cereals and vegetables."

Lord Hankey says, "It is both comprehensive and timely. A miniature and most readable encyclopaedia of what a house-wife and a pater-familias too, ought to know."

Here is an important comment from the Medical Press, which says:

"The author is primarily concerned with food as a basis for health, but, incidentally, she gives a number of recipes which should be of considerable value in the treatment of many different conditions, and which read so appetisingly that one could wish one were made the subject of such treatment without more ado . . . there is no doubt that if only more people took a comparable interest in what they eat along these lines, even at the risk of an occasional mistake, the health of the nation would be infinitely the better for it."

Mrs. Grant's book, which gives recipes for making wholemeal bread among many other things, scientifically proves that certain types of white flour are definitely poisonous. Her manuscript was read by both medical and scientific authorities and her statements verified. She acknowledges encouragement, help and information from Dr. Coghlan, Sir Robert Bristow, C.I.E., Dr. G. E. Breen, Dr. Franklin Bicknell and many others.

The next book—*Foods for good health and healing* by Dudley D'Auvergne Wright, F.R.C.S., M.R.C.S., L.R.C.P., is published by Health Science Press, Rustington, Sussex, England.

After qualifying at the University College in London, Dr. Wright had a period of study in Vienna. He became house surgeon to the London Homoeopathic Hospital and ultimately became its senior surgeon. He received the Legion of Honour (Order of Chevalier) from the French Government. He finally practised in Cape Town, South Africa as a consulting homoeopathic doctor. In his book he discusses the merits and value of vegetables and fruits in terms of healing properties, vitamins, etc. For instance this is what he says of garlic :

"Garlic has much the same properties as the onion, but its action is stronger and extends into realms somewhat outside those which concern the onion. It has the same volatile oil as the latter, and acts both on the lungs, intestinal canal and the kidneys. Its diuretic action is not, however, so marked as that of the onion, but it has a more powerful and radical action on the intestine. It more quickly removes toxic bacteria, especially bacillus proteus, and encourages the normal intestinal flora," etc., etc.

This book by Dr. Wright is really worth having.

Then there is the book by Harry Benjamin, *Your diet in health and disease*. It is published by Health for All Publishing Company, Bedford Park, Croydon, Surrey. This book went into its fourteenth impression in 1959. Read what the author says on page 38:

"How many people are aware of this debasing of the Nation's food supply, which goes on daily under our eyes to suit the ends of trade and commercialism? How many know that food is devitalised, degerminated, demineralised; bleached, chemically treated, robbed of its life-giving mineral properties, preserved and adulterated generally, without any regard being paid to its resultant effects upon men, women and children of the country?"

On page 15, he writes:

"The only way to build a healthy body is to understand *why we eat,* and *what we eat,* and once the simple fact is grasped that it is by *what we put into our mouths* that we decide either for good or evil what is to take place inside our bodies, then the way has been opened for a sane and intelligent understanding of the facts and considerations to be discussed in the present volume."

On page 18 he writes:

"The process of digestion is begun in the mouth through the medium of what is known as mastication. This is performed by teeth, assisted by the tongue and helped by a fluid secreted by the salivary glands, and known as saliva. This saliva, in addition to helping to masticate the food by making it capable of being swallowed easily, has the power to dissolve starch and turn it into a form of sugar known as maltose, by means of an enzyme or ferment known as ptyalin, which it contains. (All the digestive juices contain these enzymes or ferments; they are their active principles and have the power to change the chemical composition of the various substances taken into the body as food.) The necessity for thoroughly masticating starchy foods in the mouth, therefore will be at once apparent, as the ptyalin cannot otherwise carry out its function."

Mr. Benjamin's book is written for everyone to understand and it is a valuable contribution to health seekers.

These three books will help to educate readers in the matter of food without turning them into cranks. People just must be food conscious because of the tremendous amount of commercial contamination which breeds bad health through a gradual process. Here is an excellent example of what I mean. Take the trouble to build a small patch of compost about two feet square against a wall upon which the sun falls during the day. Throw over it a solution of bacterial compost maker which can be bought from any nursery or seed shop. Allow to mature for six weeks and then plant a couple of small tomato plants which will grow twice as quickly as those planted in ordinary earth without bacteria; twice as strong and healthy and yielding twice the volume of fruit. When the tomatoes are ripe, remove and eat without adding salt. You will get the biggest surprise of your life and will never again eat a tomato grown with artificial fertiliser unless you can help it. The compost-grown fruit is crisp, juicy and full of tantalising flavour.

CHAPTER TWELVE

SPINE ADJUSTMENT BY GRAVITATION

One of the most valuable exercises I have used at home to contribute towards good health, and still use weekly for that matter, is in adjusting the spine through suspension of the body by the head being held firm in a home-made halter. I made mine from one loaned to me by Dr. Johanna Brandt.

¹ A piece of strong canvas, doubled, must be sewn together. The length must be about two feet and the width five inches. The very ends are turned over at an angle to bring them to a point. Then a strong piece of leather is folded through a steel ring and then sewn on to each end of the canvas. The canvas is then folded in two so that the rings meet each other at one end. Then a slit, about five inches long is cut up the centre of the folded canvas—at the opposite end from the rings. When unfolded the slit will be about ten inches long in the centre of the halter. Now foam rubber, about eight inches long and two and a half inches wide must be inserted between the double layers of the canvas and stitched in or made fast by some adhesive solution. The halter is now complete.

The next step is to screw a six-inch steel hook into the centre of the framework of the door—just above your head as you stand in the open doorway. The hook must be screwed in at least two inches to be able to take a couple of hundred pounds of human weight without giving way. I have never found any difficulty with this in the average bathroom. The whole device is now ready for use after the halter has been hung on the hook in the framework by the two steel rings.

You must now stand on the floor quite erect and put your

head through the slit in the canvas with a few inches "play" under your chin, without having to take your feet off the ground. If you are too short to reach the canvas, get twelve inches of strong chain, pass it through the two steel rings and then secure the ends over the hook at a point which makes the adjustment perfect. This ensures perfect safety and no damage can be done.

The method of adjusting and loosening the spine must be gradual over a period of months. There must never be strain. In other words, at the beginning, too much weight must not be allowed to "pull" on the neck. Within three to four weeks it is a simple matter to have the full weight of the body hanging from the halter with the feet off the ground, without any danger.

To get into the halter you must stand straight and place the head between the slit in the canvas, resting your chin on the foam rubber of the front piece of canvas, and the back of your head on the other part. The ears must be pulled through the slit on either side so that they are comfortable. At this point bend the knees until you feel the head being pulled by the weight of the body, according to the amount of "bend" you have permitted with the knees. After a minute straighten the knees so that you will come back to normal without strain of any description. Rest for a couple of minutes and then do the exercise again, this time allowing a little more bending of the knees so that there is more body-weight on the halter. Do this several times and then put the halter away. It can be a daily exercise for two or three weeks at the beginning, giving more weight for the spine to carry each day, so that at the end of the period you can safely hang freely with your feet off the ground for two or three minutes at a time. Once you have managed this, the exercise should be done once a week for another month, and then only periodically, say once a month, or when there is a stiffness in the joints.

When you get to this point you will experience the tremendous advantage of this home-treatment.

The main stem of the nervous system is the spinal cord reaching the length of the trunk from the brain to the hip region. It is surrounded and protected by bony arches (neural arches) lying above the main portion of the vertebrae. The cord is a long hollow tube with a small central cavity filled with liquid—the cerebrospinal fluid. This central cavity extends upwards into the brain, where it expands into a complicated system of liquid filled sacs (ventricles). To the cord, at every segment, are attached spinal nerves which carry impulses inward from sensory structures in the skin and muscles, and outward from the cord to the muscles of the trunk and limbs. These nerves can be "pinched" between the vertebrae, making pain in certain areas unbearable, or lime or calcium can grow around them and cause all sorts of problems. I am confident that human beings were never meant to sit in offices all day or, worse, in motor cars. We are built in such a manner that exercise in moderation is essential. The compulsory tempo of our lives today makes normal, healthy living almost impossible without aids, substitutes and up-to-the-minute consciousness of the dangers which confront us. I think it is necessary for everyone to pay a monthly visit to a specialised chiropractor for spinal adjustment, but lack of time and the expense involved makes this impossible for the average person. I would like to see these practitioners install the "halter" in small cubicles so that they can attend to twenty or thirty patients at a time at a fee of not more than five shillings per visit. The alternative, of course, is the home treatment with the home-made halter and the brine bath instead of a turkish bath. Listen to what Dr. Johanna Brandt has written about the sacred spine :

"Wonders have been accomplished with the Grape Cure, but the secret of perfect physical well-being lies in the condi-

SPINE ADJUSTMENT BY GRAVITATION 93

tion of the spine. The bones should be well separated from one another by cushions of firm cartilage in order to allow an unrestricted flow of blood, nervous fluid and other vital essences from the Generator of Life, i.e. the brain, to every part of the body.

There should be no deep inward curve in the lumbar region, or "small of the back". The backbone should be straight, without being stiff. It should be pliable, supple and flexible without being limp. The full weight of the body should rest on the pelvis and be held in place by the internal muscles. This position tilts the pelvis forward and upwards, lifts the ribs, expands the chest, reduces the abdomen and straightens out that dangerous curve in the lumbar region by the pressure of which the internal organs are displaced, starved and atrophied.

No one whose pelvic bones are out of place can breathe correctly or walk gracefully. Those protruding buttocks, so conspicuous in our day, are an embarrassing warning that we have lost our balance. Every movement becomes an effort. Owing to the misuse of high heels, women and girls are the worst offenders in this respect. Since the organs of generation are the first to be affected by this loss of body harmony, the bringing forth of healthy offspring becomes an impossibility. The mothers of the race are incapacitated. Result—the decline of the body, malformations at birth, obesity, emaciation, imbecility, bald heads, eye-glasses, ear-trumpets, false teeth, cosmetics, powder and rouge.

There are many schools of physical culture teaching corrective exercises. There are trained chiropractors and osteopaths, who by the skilful manipulation of the spine, adjust the vertebrae and so release the pressure on the nerves. One and all, they serve a useful purpose. But not everyone lives within reach of a chiropractor, and many of us have not the time and energy required for the development of the body. It is a cruel fact of nature that the chronically unfit, who are in most need of physical exercise, are usually the least inclined to carry it out.

Recently something practical has been devised, a new way of straightening and lengthening the spine, a method so natural and simple, so harmless and inexpensive, and yet so amazingly effective, that a mere child can, with very little instruction, practice it at home.

By the power of gravitation the suspension of the body by the neck adjusts the whole spinal column from the base of the brain to the tip of the spine in a single movement. Naturally and painlessly something is accomplished in five seconds that physical exercise fails to do in so many years.

A stiff spine does not yield its full length immediately, and herein lies the safety of the student. There is no danger of straining ligaments, rupturing veins or otherwise injuring the delicate membranes and nerves of the spine when the exercise is done carefully. This method of adjusting the spine is slow because it is natural; the improvement in health is gradual and steady, but its benefits reveal themselves in many ways from the first moment of its adoption.

This gentle stretching of the spine can never injure anyone. If at first it seems to have injurious effects, this is due to the stirring up of poisons by the unwonted exercise and stimulation of the circulation. There is a new rush of blood to the affected parts; one experiences a delightful, warm glow at first, after which a soothing sense of rest and relaxation. When the spine is normal these sensations are absent; or the spine may have become so stiff that the exercise has no apparent effect. In either case, continuing the hanging-exercise can never be anything but beneficial, because it will effectually prevent the normal spine from becoming stiff, and by its gentle action it is bound in time to relieve the condition of the stiff spine to some extent and prevent it from getting worse. When unusual symptoms occur such as a feeling of pins-and-needles, soreness or rheumatic pains, it is advisable to discontinue the exercise for a few days, or to modify them. Remember that every sign of discomfort is an indication of the presence of poisons. *The hanging exercise alone will not avail to remove them.* The Grape Cure; fasting or a special fruit diet are necessary.

The idea has got abroad that when the spine is out of alignment the bones are out of place. This is impossible. Only a violent wrench or shock could displace the vertebrae, and in that case the injury done to the spinal cord would be so great that instant death would be the result. What actually happens is that there is an undue muscular contraction on one side of the spine which causes an undue relaxation of the muscles on the other side. Contracted muscles mean congested nerves. Acute pain may be the result. Continued contraction will cause chronic spinal lesions, and these will in time cause what is known as disease in the organs to which they are related."

Dr. Johanna Brandt warns that there is a certain danger of overstraining the ligaments if the exercise is overdone, and this, of course, applies to any kind of exercise.

CHAPTER THIRTEEN

THE DANGER OF CERTAIN BEVERAGES

It is common knowledge that coffee, especially in large quantities, is very bad for one. The same applies to tea and cocoa, but I think it would be a mistake to become crankish about these things, since everything in moderation is good. The body is designed to excrete toxins and this job it will always do provided it is not abused too much. What I am very convinced about is what is known as "cold drinks", more especially for the sake of small children. You will understand my anxiety in this respect after you have read what Professor Douw. G. Steyn, Professor of Pharmacology, Medical Faculty, University of Pretoria, South Africa, has to say, and he is acknowledged as one of the foremost toxicologists in the world. He writes :

"The fact (a) that some of the cool drinks contained appreciable quantities of caffeine, organic and inorganic acids and synthetic dyes; (b) that many complaints of severe gastric irritation are received from individuals who consumed these caffein-containing cool drinks, and (c) that these drinks were being consumed in enormous quantities by children and even toddlers and babies, prompted the author to investigate their possible harmful and carcinogenic effects, for which he received a grant from the South African Council for Individual and Scientific Research. The experiments were planned in such a way that the effects of a ration deficient in Vitamin A and B complex could be compared with those of a ration containing all the essential nutrients. Three hundred and sixty young rats were employed in the experiments which ran for seventeen months. The rats were permitted to consume the cool drink daily or on alternate days at the rate of approximate 25/50 cc/kg bodyweight daily. This is equivalent to a child, 30 kg in weight, consuming $3\frac{3}{4}$ to $7\frac{1}{2}$ bottles (each 200 cc) of cool drink daily. An important point to be considered is that the rats had food ad lib, and that children, more often than not, consume large quantities of cool drink on an empty stomach. Each batch of cool drink was chemically analysed and the biological effects on the rats reflected the nature and the quantity of the ingredients. The different batches of the cool drink yielded different results according to the nature and quantities of the ingredients present. This was also reflected in variation in the taste of the beverage. At the termination of the experiments all the surviving experimental animals, including the controls, were killed and specimens for histological examination collected but not yet fully examined. In the meantime the following remarks may be made : (a) Diet played a most important rôle in the susceptibility of the rats to the harmful effects of the cool drink. Protein and vitamin deficiency caused a most pronounced increase in the susceptibility to the harmful effects of the beverage." (A young rat living on a ration deficient in protein and vitamin A and B complex, and receiving the cool drink daily was shown in a photograph which also featured a picture of the control rat receiving only the deficient ration and no cool drink, and it is twice the size. It must be emphasised that each rat was eating the same diet.)

Professor Steyn goes on to say :

"If we were to apply the results obtained upon rats to human beings, we would begin to realise more and more to what extent the under-privileged and under-nourished, especially children, who live so extensively on white bread and cool drinks suffer from the effects of the presence of appreciable quantities of undesirable and harmful ingredients of some cool drinks. An important aspect of the cool drink trade in hot and dry climates is the enormous quantity consumed. The experimental rats consumed approximately twice to four times the quantities of cool drink that children in the Republic of South Africa do. The animals preferred cool drink to water. (*b*) The cool drinks had harmful effects on the young rats in that it caused *Alopecia*, general weakness, paresis, pronounced retarded growth and loss in condition, tooth caries and early death. Autopsy revealed *petechiae* in the gastric mucosa, and small gastric ulcers were very prevalent. The department of health should exercise strict control over the cool drink trade. It is essential that all the ingredients of cool drinks offered for sale to the public, and the quantities of the ingredients, should be registered with the Department of Health, and that if they were permitted to contain caffeine, the quantities should be disclosed on the label."

Professor Steyn's report is a terrible indictment. Parents should heed this warning.

It would be wrong to condemn any particular cool drink because of this analysis, as some could be quite harmless, but because of colouring matter and the use of certain toxic chemicals, they could also be harmful. *It is the duty of Women's Organisations throughout the world to insist that all foodstuffs and beverages made with doubtful ingredients, should be analysed, and the findings published in national newspapers.*

There is absolutely no reason why drinks made from fresh fruits should not take the place of the synthetic product, with equal profit to the bottling companies. Is the status of human flesh and blood so insignificant that it is now merely a pawn in the game of profit-making? It would seem so. Is man now without the human dignity and initiative given him to protect his person? I don't believe it. In many cases—more particularly with cigarette advertising—commerce has turned people into common slaves, but the time will come when common sense, honesty, courage and particularly unity, will make the world a better place to live in. People must get together and condemn products which are harmful.

Sugar and salt. Excessive quantities of these are also dangerous. Professor Steyn says that ordinary table salt taken in excessive quantities over long periods, damages and weakens the small blood vessels (capillaries) and possibly the kidneys. This, he says, leads not only to the accummulation of fluid (oedema) in various parts of the body, but such weakened capillaries also rupture easily (apoplexy). It is calculated that we ingest twice to three times more salt that our bodies need. Professor Steyn says that there is a concensus of opinion among nutritionists that we, and especially our children, daily ingest quantities of sugar far in excess of our needs. It is ingested in the form of many sweetened foods, candy, jam, preserves, cool drinks and other beverages, cakes, etc. Even infants are taught to like the taste of sugar by dipping their dummies in sugar or sugared water, and older children are enticed to eat their food by adding masses of sugar to it. In this way our children are being taught from their earliest childhood to want everything sweetened. Professor Steyn says that excessive quantities of sugar affect our health in various ways, namely :

(1) Sugar favours the development of gastrointestinal catarrh, gastric ulcers, chronic indigestion, appendicitis and gall bladder disease.

(2) Under certain conditions oxalic acid is formed from sugar present in the intestinal tract and this leads to the formation of kidney and bladder stones.

(3) Best and his colleagues (*British Medical Journal* No. 5, 1959, pp. 1001–1006) proved that rats ingesting large quantities of sugar develop liver disease (accumulation of fat in the liver and subsequent development of cirrhosis [hardening] of the liver). This effect of the inges-

tion of excessive quantities of sugar is due to the fact that, through lack of appetite, nutritious foods containing the so-called lipotropic factors, choline and methionine, which prevent the accumulation of fat in the liver, are ingested in insufficient quantities.

(4) *Tooth caries.* Professor Steyn says that there can be no doubt that the constant eating of candy, especially sticky sweets, cake, etc., and the excessive drinking of acid cool drinks are two of the most important causes of the very prevalent tooth decay in the modern child and in many adults. I agree with Toverud (*British Dental Journal*, Vol. 86, 1949, p. 191) when he emphasises the importance of a good calcifying diet and the minimal use of sugar as sweets or sweet cakes. He deprecates the habit, so common among mothers, of dipping dummies in sugared water, honey or rose-hip syrup, and of giving "suckable" sweets in the first year of life, as it certainly leads to the most undesirable and harmful habit of wanting all foods sweetened and the constant eating of sweets and cakes, which also impair the appetite for wholesome foods at meals. It should therefore be realised, says Professor Steyn, that excessive consumption of sugar causes tooth decay, not only by providing conditions in the mouth favourable to the multiplication of acidogenic bacteria but also because, through lack of appetite for wholesome food, it impairs the ingestion of the building stones of sound teeth (calcium, phosphorus, etc.).

Profesor Steyn says of the ingestion of excessive amounts of carbohydrates, the presence of incompletely oxidised products of sugar and other carbohydrates in the blood and tissues, is probably responsible to a large extent for headaches, including migraine, increased susceptibility to infections (colds, sinusitis, tonsillitis, bronchitis), etc., and the very prevalent allergic diseases (hay fever, asthma, skin infections), etc.

CHAPTER FOURTEEN

COOKING UTENSILS

For many years doctors and nature-cure specialists have warned me against cooking food in aluminium utensils, but I was never given a valid reason for it.

Professor Steyn's article on cool drinks appears in a booklet with details of research on the possible danger of contamination to food when cooked in certain utensils.

The article under the heading of *Food and Beverages in relation to cancer* was presented before the Symposium of Potential Cancer Hazards from Chemical Additives to Foodstuffs, held by the International Union against Cancer in Rome on 10th August to the 21st, 1956. It reads: "Betts[57] states that according to his 'experiences and observations', metal poisoning, including aluminium, has been noticed to cause gastric diseases, and also cancer. Information on this aspect of aluminium poisoning is, however, very meagre and incomplete."

During World War II experiments were conducted by the author (Professor Steyn) upon dogs with food cooked in aluminium pots. Those animals, except the controls, were fed on meat and porridge cooked in aluminium pots. One group received meat cooked in an alkaline medium (sodium bicarbonate) and one group, meat cooked in an acid medium (vinegar). The dogs which received meat cooked in the alkaline medium developed symptoms of chronic poisoning within four to six months, viz lack of appetite, loss in weight, constipation and apathy. One of the animals died after eight months and autopsy revealed a severe chronic gastroenteritis. From examination of the aluminium pots it was evident that an

alkaline medium causes much more severe corrosion of the
pots than an acid medium.

In view of the extensive use of aluminium cooking utensils
and the pronounced corrosion caused by alkaline media, it is
most important to establish without doubt whether there is
a possibility of danger in their use. It is obvious that in the
execution of such investigations a large number of factors
should be taken into consideration. The fact that Dr. Joseph
Gillman, Professor of Physiology, University of the Witwaters-
rand, Johannesburg, South Africa, had found the gall-bladder
contents of many corpses heavily contaminated with aluminium, lends greater significance to the problem of chronic
aluminium poisoning. In what way did this aluminium find
its way into the system? Through food, beverages, drinking
water or drugs?

That ends the article of Professor Steyn which gave me the
urge to a great deal of thought, and then, quite out of the
blue I remembered an experience I had on my farm with my
dogs.

I was breeding Harlequin Great Danes but lost three of my
champions from enteritis and the veterinary surgeon just could
not give me a reason for this malady. I also lost an entire litter
on one occasion for the same reason. Years later, after reading
Professor Steyn's article my thoughts turned to the method in
which I cooked the animals' food. It was in aluminium—
nothing but aluminium! It is quite reasonable for me to link
the death of my animals with aluminium poisoning, after
all the warnings I have had from doctors not to cook in that
medium; after reading the article, and after an experience I
had quite recently with a friend. He was constantly suffering
from enteritis, until one day I challenged him on the medium
of his wife's cooking utensils. They were aluminium! Naturally I told him the story of the dogs, and the article by Professor Steyn which was enough to prompt him to cook in
enamel. I am glad to say that there is no more enteritis in
that family. Recently, too, one of my staff developed open

wounds on her right ankle which refused to heal even after a great deal of treatment by her doctors. I enquired the nature of her beverage intake and discovered it to be largely coffee and cool drinks. I suggested that she discontinued both. Within a week her condition improved considerably without medical treatment, but the abscess just would not heal properly. I then discovered that aluminium pots were being used for the family cooking. I described how corrosion took place and that the small particles of aluminium entered the body through the food and brought about poisoning. Naturally all aluminium utensils were withdrawn from the kitchen. At the end of another week the wound had completely and permanently healed. It was quite magical.

Let me make it quite clear that I have neither the moral nor the legal right to condemn aluminium for cooking purposes, but in the circumstances it is my unquestionable duty to suggest to people who constantly suffer from any form of enteritis to withdraw these utensils from the kitchen for a sufficient period to make a proper test. If they are found to be the cause of the poisoning, these utensils must never again be used for actual cooking, but there is no possible harm, I should think, if they were used for storage purposes. Again, I suggest that prominent Women's Organisations should urge Governments to condemn all foods and cooking utensils, whatever they may be made of, if they can be proved to be injurious to health. Women have been known to give their very lives for their children. Is it too much to ask that they give a little thought and energy towards a system which is undermining the health of nations?

CHAPTER FIFTEEN

MENTAL ASPECTS OF HEALTH

People like myself who have spent the major part of their lives in an environment of illness, inevitably grow a sharper sense of balance and observation after they have been freed from their life-long burden. It is then not difficult to recognise most things in their proper perspective and to approach them with a pattern of positive thought and action—hence the writing of this book!

Those unfortunate people who are still burdened, tend to allow their illness to inflict untold damage to their minds and bodies through fear, and who can blame them when there is no help from the medical profession for so-called incurable diseases, and when hope begins to dwindle? Was I not myself a complete example of this state of affairs? Of course I was, but I emerged not only with a permanent cure, but also with the *knowledge that only the thing a man fears can destroy him and that fear of any description is wholly unnecessary in anyone's life!*

In retrospect it is obvious that my own sickness-pattern was always influenced by frustration—a very potent off-shoot of fear. Had I been capable of shedding the bonds of inhibition at that time, and clothed myself in the freshness of truth and fearlessness, Mr. McDonagh's treatment would have given me health-balance and happiness for the rest of my life, because, like the grape treatment, his was one of elimination without drugs. Now that my thought pattern is positive and fearless as a result of the grape treatment and the spiritual elevation I have been privileged to enjoy, I recognise the body for what it is—a temporary vehicle to transport the soul through yet another passage of time. I also recognise that each one of us is divided into three distinct and separate units—each powerful in its own right—but wholly destructive unless united—and that there are seven stages of life on earth and beyond it!

The first is the stratum of mineral life beneath the earth in its concentrated, vibrant and sometimes very destructive forms. The second stratum is the beautiful carpet of vegetation which covers the earth in all its glory, and the waters of the exotic little streams; the rivers and the mighty oceans, also destructive in moments of imbalance. The third stratum or stage of life is made up of the birds, the beasts, the insects and the microbes and all the life which feeds on the vegetation and lives in the waters. The law governing this life is the law of the jungle! It too can be devastating!

Then comes the fourth stratum. Man! Inhibited man in all his self-made glory—knowing only the power of his own will and self-created vanity, creating laws for his own selfish purpose. His life pattern is also destructive because it is governed by fear. Man who claims the right to indiscriminate killing, but strangely enough, in his fourth stratum he is justified. He is justified because he knows no other law.

His God is the god of gold and his power is that of greed, excitement and self-indulgence. He is without mental balance although there are times when he proves himself to be brilliant and inspiring among those in his own stratum. His body is without balance and his mind is like a rapier covered with rust, poisoning the wounds of each thrust. He will always survive until he destroys himself!

Then there is the life of man in the fifth stratum, on earth.

Nearly two thousand years ago a man was born into our world with a message of truth which he delivered faithfully until he was crucified physically by those in the fourth stratum who feared him. He had explained that every human being on earth was endowed with a Spirit, a part of the Living God who created the world—a part of the true eternal life. Some of his words were simple so that all could understand; others were parabolic for the mystics to interpret—more especially on occasions when greater inspiration came their way. The man they called Jesus Christ made it abundantly clear that unless we allowed our spirit to awaken and flow naturally and unhindered towards its counterpart which is God—naming Him their Father, there would be no real vision; no real strength; no real courage or understanding, and no possible hope! He also said that there would be no health or joy! In His parabolic message he spoke of the trinity of man's body and his mind and his spirit as being the wholeness, the richness and the balance—the perfect equilibrium! He preached the need for the elevation of the Spirit, which, pure, whole and indestructible, awakens and thrives only on constant prayer—daily prayer—preferably in the House of God, thus uniting the mind, the body and the spirit, when, for the first time in his life man becomes aware of perfection; the dimension which frees him from the domination of his ego and tears away his roots of fear, frustration, inhibition, anger and all forms of violence in thought, word and deed—even to the destruction of the smallest insect—necessary though it may seem. He spoke of the real purpose of living on this earth —that of constant purification in all things, counter-balancing original sin and its escalations; drawing man into the fifth stratum where he would discover truth, wisdom, fearlessness, the simplest faith and the deepest knowledge, and that these attributes would become second nature, directing him through the paths of love, kindness, beauty, and selflessness, so that when death comes on this earth it will be the moment when grace and beauty adorns the soul on its journey through that mighty span 'twixt God and Man into the sixth stratum for further purification, so that in the end it may go unto and into the Kingdom of God—the Seventh Stratum!

CHAPTER SIXTEEN

SUMMARY

I discovered so much because I was in such great need. Inspiration came in many ways to me. I will always believe that it was the will of God that guided me to treat myself with the grapes, and to write this record of my discovery. Looking back in retrospect it becomes only too obvious that the only treatment on earth for illness is through ELIMINATION; a process of reducing the toxic content in the body very gradually, so that the body can heal itself. It must always be remembered that severe illness such as cancer rarely grows overnight. It takes time to breed and to manifest itself, but it can also unbreed, if I may use that word, through a gradual process of self-purification of the body, through elimination; and the mind through faith and the exercise and communion of prayer, so that the spirit, whole, pure and incorruptible can take charge again in its mystery of creating wholeness.

I pray with all my heart that doctors will start experimenting with the grape treatment for every known illness. It does take courage to get away from synthetic drugs which really don't heal at all (since only the body can do this) and practice natural cures, but there will be a beginning, because several doctors have already told me quite openly that they do not believe in the system of drugs for healing, and that they are sick unto death of the whole business. I have treated several doctors with the grape cure and they have testified in no uncertain manner to its magical healing power.

It would be stupid to condemn modern medicine as a

whole, or the progress which surgery has made in the last few decades, but unless they are allied to a natural, normal and gradual healing process provided by nature, it will not be many years before illness as such and the ability to cope with it gets completely out of hand. It is essential that the human body gets a periodical, natural treatment to free the blood-stream and organs of their destructive toxic elements. There are seven natural doctors to draw from for this purpose. The fasting cure; water treatments applied externally and internally; the ice cure; the liquid diet which comprises all fruit and vegetable juices, honey drinks, etc.; the exclusive grape treatment; the fruit cure consisting of uncooked fruits and vegetables, dried fruits, honey, nuts, etc.; and finally deep breathing which includes spine treatment, manipulations, massage, etc.

Sleeplessness can be cured by taking a tablespoonful of honey in a glass of water, or preferably diluted bottled pure grape juice. Sleep will come within fifteen to twenty minutes after taking the draught. I would like to end my story with one or two quotations from a very small book, but indeed a gem of literature entitled *As man thinketh,* by James Allen, published by Fowler and Co., 29 Ludgate Hill, London, E.C., but which can also be obtained from *The Bookworm* in Hertford, Herts., England. On pages 26–27 he writes: "Disease and health like circumstances, are 'rooted in thought'. Sickly thoughts will express themselves through a sickly body. Thoughts of fear have been known to kill a man as speedily as a bullet, and they are continually killing thousands of people just as surely, though less rapidly. The people who live in fear of disease are the people who get it. Anxiety quickly demoralises the whole body and lays it open to the entrance of disease; while impure thoughts, even if not physically indulged, will soon shatter the nervous system.

Strong, pure and happy thoughts build up the body in vigour and grace.

The body is a delicate and plastic instrument which responds readily to the thoughts by which it is impressed, and habits of thoughts will produce their own effects, good or bad, upon it. Man will continue to have impure and poisoned blood, so long as they propagate impure thoughts. Out of a clean heart comes a clean life and a clean body. Out of a defiled mind proceeds a defiled life and a corrupt body. Thought is the fount of action, life and manifestation; make the fountain pure and all will be pure. Change of diet will not help a man who will not change his thoughts. When a man makes his thoughts pure, he no longer desires impure food. Clean thoughts make clean habits. The so-called Saint who does not wash his body is not a Saint. He who has strengthened and purified his thoughts does not need to consider the malevolent microbe. If you would protect your body, guard your mind. If you would renew your body, beautify your mind. Thoughts of malice, envy, disappointment, despondency, rob the body of its health and grace. A sour face does not come by chance; it is made by sour thoughts. Wrinkles that mar are drawn by folly, passion and pride. I know a woman of ninety-six who has the bright, innocent face of a girl. I know a man well under middle age whose face is drawn into inharmonious contours. The one is the result of a sweet and sunny disposition; the other is the outcome of passion and discontent". That ends the excerpt from Mr. Allen's book, but I must tell you about Master Tara Singh, the 76-year-old leader of the Sikh people in the Punjab, who went on a 48-day fast only half a dozen years ago. It was in protest of what he considered an injustice to his people. It was his selflessness and spiritual strength which protected him from fear and made his fast successful. It was incidental that his family doctors afterwards proclaimed the lengthening of his life-span by ten years, because the fast had rid him of all the illnesses from which he had been suffering—but it proved that when the spirit is strong, all things are possible.

Pure minds and healthy bodies are the most treasured possessions on earth; all of us should plan to build them for ourselves, and for our children, maintaining them in a state of permanent radiance with the power, beauty and harmony of the living spirit in communion with God, and it is on this note that my story ends.

DR. JOHANNA BRANDT

Before leaving London in December 1956, I was given a letter to a naturopath in Capetown. I made my visit before starting the grape treatment, but she was away. Four weeks later, after my successful cure, I again visited her. Imagine my tremendous pleasure and surprise, when, after relating the story of my illness, my experiment upon myself with the grapes, and my miraculous cure, she went quietly to her bookshelf and withdrew a small volume which she presented to me. It was called *The Grape Cure*—for cancer and other diseases—by Johanna Brandt, N.D., Ph.N., M.A., who wrote it thirty years previously, after having cured herself of abdominal cancer by the grape diet. What a remarkable coincidence! Naturally, I showed anxiety to meet her, which I did after the termination of my own treatment three weeks later. Dr. Johanna Brandt was a remarkable old lady (she has since died, I regret to say) who, I am happy to relate, became a staunch and lovable friend. She was hale and hearty on her eighty-fifth birthday, with not one of her faculties impaired, and she was still visiting and treating patients with the magical grape. Very graciously she gave me written permission to make quotations from her book to substantiate my own. Her book is undoubtedly an inspired classic, brilliantly and very beautifully written from her heart. Unquestionably a copy should be in every home because it is full of wisdom, and truth, and it goes into minute detail about how to get well and keep well all your life! The book—*The Grape Cure*—can be obtained in Afrikaans or English from one of Dr. Johanna

Brandt's daughters, Mrs. E. Kellerman, 87A H. van Rensburg Street, Pietersburg, Transvaal, South Africa.

The introduction to the book is by the famous American doctor and naturopath, Dr. Benedict Lust, M.D., N.D., who wrote :

"It is a great privilege to pay tribute to that great woman and healer, Johanna Brandt, on the appearance of the eighth edition of her work, *The Grape Cure*. It was my privilege to introduce her to America a number of years ago, and for her service to humanity, the American School of Naturopathy also offered her its official recognition for the great work she is doing for humanity. *The Grape Cure* has continued to help suffering man for several decades, and it is my earnest hope that Johanna Brandt's name and work will continue to bring relief to those who need it. The successive printings of her book, of which this is the eighth, prove the merit of the system which she expounded so many years ago."

AUTHOR'S PREFACE—1928

Dr. Johanna Brandt commences her book thus :

"In the present desperate need of the world I am offering this book of instruction as my contribution towards a solution of the great problem which is known as the cancer scourge.

It would be wrong to raise false hopes in the mind of the afflicted. Merely eating grapes will not cure cancer. There is far more to it than that. The poisons that are stirred up by the chemical action of the grape must be eliminated, and this is done by the methods of natural healing which I have endeavoured to explain in these pages. It is my duty to state emphatically that very few cases that have reached the final stages of the dread disease can be saved. The condition is relieved, suffering is mitigated to an almost incredible extent, but there is no time for the purification of the blood, which is the first essential in arresting the course of the disease.

Under favourable circumstances, far advanced cases of cancer have been cured by us; that is to say, when they have not been touched by the surgeon's knife. When, apart from the degenerating action of the virulent cancer poisons, the nerves have been severed and there is a permanent interruption in the circulation, and the flow of nervous and other life forces; when organs and glands have been removed, limbs amputated; the blood poisoned by injections, and the tissues destroyed by the use of radium and electricity. When patients come to us in this state there is nothing left except the shell to work on, then, I repeat, the Grape and Nature Cure do not avail to save them. Much of our information is based on personal experience and observation, but we have also drawn from the best recognised sources in the fields of drugless healing in England, America, Europe, and in fact every part of the world. To the inspired authors of many valuable works we owe a debt of gratitude that can never be paid. The list of their names is too long to be enumerated here, but we shall always be pleased to supply our readers with any information they may require."

"THE STORY OF THE DISCOVERY"

by Johanna Brandt
which appeared in the New York Evening Graphic *on*
January 21st 1928

"I was born in the heart of South Africa in 1876. Over fifty years ago my forefathers were heavy meat-eaters, and practically lived on game, as did most South Africans in those days. I do not know whether this has anything to do with the fact that cancer is the greatest scourge of our country, but I think so. There was a lot of cancer in my father's family, and my mother died of cancer in 1916. The doctors tell us that the disease is not hereditary. This may be true but the pre-disposing causes of cancer in my mother's body may have been present in my own. It is not unreasonable to assume this. Be that as it may, as long as I can remember, I suffered from gastric attacks, bilious trouble and stomach ulcers. It is cruel when one is of an highly romantic temperament, to have to turn one's internal organs inside out for public inspection. Why could it not have been something less prosaic? Heart disease, lung trouble or a delicate throat? But a stomach! A reeking, fermenting stomach, and a blatantly conscious one at that!

After the anguishing spectacle of my mother's martyrdom, I had one shock after another. National, family and other troubles. Life became a ghastly nightmare, and through it all I was conscious of a gnawing pain at the left side of my stomach. Cancer? I was not afraid of it. In my ignorance I thought I had reached the limit of human endurance. I saw in cancer a possible release.

A friend, meeting my husband one day, inquired after my health, and was so struck by his reply that she repeated it to me: 'What must I say about my wife? The hope of death is keeping her alive, and fear of life is nearly killing her.' The *hope of death*. That was it. But I was puzzled to know how my secret had been discovered. My plan of action was carefully pre-arranged. I would allow nothing to be done that would prolong life. If it was really cancer, no medicines would be taken to check the disease. No injections. No drugs to alleviate pain. And, under no circumstances, the application of the surgeon's knife.

At this time a little book was put into my hands. *The fasting cure* by Upton Sinclair. It thrilled me. A new hope surged through me—the hope of relief from suffering. Here was something that appealed to my common sense—something constructive—a nature cure. The book set the fasting ball rolling in our house. I fasted for seven days.

The result was disappointing. Nothing daunted I fasted again and persuaded everyone else to fast. In time I set up a fasting business—free of charge. Anyone and everyone could fast for nothing under my supervision. I became highly experienced and cured everyone but myself.

The study of one system of healing led to another. Our home was stacked with the best American books and magazines on the science of spinal adjustment; German water cures; Swiss sunbathing; Russian fruit cures, and Oriental works on the science of deep breathing.

A flame had been lit which nothing could extinguish. It was my joy and privilege to see our large family of sons and daughters growing up tall, strong and athletic. I once overheard the following fragment of a good-humoured argument between two small sons : 'You talk more nonsense in a day than Charlie Chaplin in a week. Eat more fruit, man. You will feel much better.' 'Fruit? What you want is a jolly good fast.'

We Fletcherised raw carrots and peanuts until our jaws ached. We began the day with spinal exercises and finished it by sleeping outside. The whole family joined hands with me in the campaign against disease. Our fortune was spent in building up a system of natural healing so perfect in its simplicity and economy that it would meet the needs of the farming population in the remotest regions of South Africa. I wrote books and answered thousands of letters, but under it all I knew that my own internal trouble was not responding to nature cure.

'Nine year battle for life'

My battle for life lasted nine years. I fasted myself to a skeleton. I fasted beyond starvation point, which is a most unusual proceeding, consuming my own life tissues in the effort to destroy the growth. With every fast the growth was unmistakably checked. But it was not destroyed. On the contrary it seemed to take a new hold of me whenever I broke the fast—*because I took the wrong foods afterwards!*

'How cancer thrives'

I knew exactly what was taking place. I knew that it was wrong to undermine the system by injurious fasting and then to nourish the growth by wrong feeding. What was I to do? There was no one to advise me, but while experimenting on myself I was learning something new every day. *Among other things, I learned that cancer thrives on every form of animal food—the more impure the better!*

I suffered from horrible and disgusting cravings for blood—for beef and rich blood sausages, for stimulating and highly seasoned foods. The growth was now pushing its way through the diaphragm towards the heart and left lung. I seemed to see it like a red octopus feeding on the impure blood at the base of the lung. Breathing became difficult. I spat blood occasionally. One night in August 1920, I had a terrible attack of vomiting and purging, with excruciating pain. Towards morning I brought up a quantity of half-digested blood.

'In serious condition'

Matters were becoming serious. The thought of the death certificate and possible complications troubled me. I sent for our family physician. He ordered me to lie still in bed for three months. Under his supervision I fasted twelve days. Plenty of time now to write glowing accounts of the wonder of nature cure to distant correspondents. More than ever I realised the importance of saving my own life in order to convince and save others. It was under this fast that I first noticed an ominous sign—the presence of digested blood—known in medical circles as 'coffee grounds' in the stools after the use of an enema. Still more disconcerting was to find that I no longer put on weight on breaking the fast.

Towards the end of 1920 I seemed to be fasting chronically, four days, seven, ten, and finally three weeks in December.

Nothing has been said in this article about the mental aspect of healing. The subject is too big. It forms the most wonderful story of my life, but I must now be content to state that I became superconscious. I had 'unerring hunches', and cultivated a bowing acquaintance with my sublimal self—whatever that may be.

All this fasting brought about a slight improvement and I somehow dragged through 1921. Then in November I was persuaded by my doctor to go into the General Hospital in Johannesburg for an x-ray examination. The reader will find an account of this on page 223 of my book on the fasting cure.

Many plates were taken, and a noted surgeon pronounced his verdict—the stomach was being divided into two by a vicious fibrous growth. An immediate operation was recommended as the only means of prolonging my life.

Dr. W. Stewart who was operating in the X-ray Department, was much interested in my experience, and invited me to his house for another x-ray examination, if I found myself still in the land of the living in six months. Encouraged by this mark of sympathy, I fasted three weeks in December, drinking pure water and lying in the morning sun. When after six months I went under the x-rays again, no trace of the growth could be found!

'But pain remained'

I assured the doctors, however, that the pain was still there, and told them that I was looking for a food which would answer a three-fold purpose, viz., destroy the growth effectually; eliminate the poison, and build new tissue.

The three years that followed were years of great

suffering, but I kept on fasting and dieting alternatively, and in 1925, after a seven day fast, I accidentally discovered a food that had the miraculous effect of healing me completely within six weeks.

The publication of this discovery will be of more value after the particulars set forth in this article have been proved to be facts.

I therefore call upon the Medical Council to have an exploratory operation performed. The gravity of the disease can only be estimated by an examination of the extent of damage done, and then only can the efficacy of the cure be established.

A method which will cure cancer will cure almost any other disease. While I was experimenting on myself I was often discouraged by the thought that very few people would be able to undergo such rigorous treatment. Even the perusal of these harrowing details would plunge the reader into a state of fear and doubt, but it is the sum total of my experience that I hope to bring before the public. All that prolonged fasting was unnecessary. The mistakes I made need not be made by other patients. Our system of healing has been greatly modified by the discovery of the food cure. And while the patient is undergoing the cure, for his or her own partciular complaint, nature is secretly restoring and rejuvenating every part of the body. The senses become abnormally acute; dim eyes brighten; faded hair takes on new gloss; the lifeless, hopeless voice becomes vibrant, magnetic, and the complexion clears.

I have seen beautiful sets of teeth loose in their suppurating sockets, become steady and fixed within a few weeks; the gums free of pyorrhoea within a few months.

I have watched old people getting young, and young people becoming superbly beautiful, *and with every new, entrancing revelation of the* WONDERS OF NATURE CURE,

I have dedicated my life anew to this joyous work of spreading the good news."

Dr. Johanna Brandt goes on to say that from the Medical Fraternity there was no response to her challenge, although a doctor and surgeon of exceptionally high standing called and encouraged her to remain steadfast in her plan for natural healing, which is exactly what she did.

She tells in her book about doctors who actually experimented with the Grape Cure for her cancer patients, and whilst some who had undergone serious operations succumbed under her treatment, others are still living in spite of the havoc wrought by the surgeon's knife. For instance, a young woman living on Coney Island who had undergone eight operations on the rectum and the base of the spine for cancer. With one exception, this was one of the most remarkable cases cured by the grapes. Dr. Brandt says that she had never seen anyone so completely poisoned and mutilated. Under the grape diet (and the patient continued it longer than other patients) the pus poured from her.

When she began to pass worms Dr. Brandt knew that the patient's ordeal was nearly over, as the grape chemicals ferret out the most deep-seated cause of the trouble, and drives it out of the system. The patient's life was a perpetual martyrdom. The coccyx had been removed, and she could never again sit properly, and nothing could relieve the excruciating pain in the spine, but, she says, "to look upon that transfigured face, fills one with awe". The eyes shone with an unearthly beauty; her skin was soft and smooth—like the petals of a rose. Sanctified by suffering this woman had emerged from the abyss of premature death to be a witness to the divine healing properties of the grape.

Dr. Johanna Brandt writes this of another patient :

"We had a 'star' patient in the Bronx—a middle-aged woman—the mother of a large family. When first I was

called to her she was in the final stages of cancer of the
stomach and bowels, vomiting night and day! When this
stage has been reached it is not wise to begin a drastic
cure—but that death chamber was charged with so much
filial love and passionate anxiety, that I had not the heart
to refuse my services. Just a few grapes were administered
at a time. Within twenty-four hours the vomiting stopped.
The desperate strain was relieved. But the emaciated
victim went steadily down, passing through all the phases
of debility and weakness until she actually reached the
unconscious stage. The grim struggle for life lasted nearly
two months. One healing crisis succeeded another. Finally,
her legs began to swell. 'This is the end,' one of her sons
whispered. 'Yes,' I replied, 'this is the end of the cure,
the poisons have now been collected in a safe place. Wrap
these swollen limbs up in grape compresses diluted with
water. Open the pores. In a day or two—tomorrow—the
swellings will have subsided.' *Tomorrow* had a distinct
improvement in the condition, and soon no trace was left
of the dropsical symptoms.

Wonder to relate, the hard mass in the ascending colon
had been disappearing gradually. Nothing was left of that,
and the stomach was now so pure and strong, that the
patient's incessant demand was for food.

At this point I must make special mention of the fact
that during the most critical period, when the patient was
no longer able to take grapes, the pure juice of the grapes
was administered with a spoon every ten or fifteen minutes.
This natural stimulant tided her over the supreme crisis.
I am quite sure she could not have been saved in any other
way. As she grew stronger she drank grape juice by the
pint, and gradually other fruits were added to the menu.
She is now able to indulge in a delicious variety of raw
salads, a dish of sliced tomatoes with olive oil, a ripe banana
mashed with sour cream, and her favourite beverage,
buttermilk."

Dr. Brandt continues:

"Some other test cases have passed through experiences no less remarkable. In research work the most satisfactory experiments may be made with external cancer. While the system is being drained of its poisons under the grape diet, the wounds are kept open with frequent applications of grape poultices, compresses or fomentations. The discharge from these wounds in the early stages of the treatment is horrible in the extreme. As nature works very thoroughly, the discharge may continue for weeks; the grape chemicals eat their way deeper and deeper into the diseased flesh, and the wounds do not heal until all the poisons have been eliminated. *Then the healing proceeds from within.* No scabs or crusts are formed, as long as the wounds are kept moist, but from the glistening bone outwards, the process of reconstruction is carried on. Healthy, rosy granulations of new flesh appear, and gradually the cavities are filled up. With such miraculous evidences that a certain cure for cancer has been found, one is filled with a new enthusiasm."

Under the heading of:

"THE SECRET OF THE SUCCESS OF THE GRAPE CURE",

Dr. Johanna Brandt continues:

"Apart from the rich organic sugar in the grapes, the fact that they contain proteins, the great body builders, partially explains why new tissue is built with such extraordinary rapidity on an exclusively grape diet. But science has not yet discovered what elements in the grape break down the malignant growths. Some fine essence, which has hitherto escaped observation, must be present in this *Queen of fruits.* Perhaps this elusive substance will be found in the pure distilled water of the grape. We are only on the threshold of our discoveries and experiments, learning something new every day. Diluted, it is used for cleaning the throat, ears, nose and mouth; applied externally on wounds in the form of poultices and compresses; diluted with water and introduced per rectum as food.

But let us see what can be achieved by the grape diet only, without these supplementary methods.

The mono diet. (One food only.) *It was the exclusive grape diet that saved my life in the end. After the nine years battle with death, I discovered accidentally that fresh grapes, when taken alone, answered the three requirements of solving, eliminating and building.*

Like everyone else I had been eating grapes for years. I grew up among the Vineyards of South Africa, and the finest grapes in the world were to be found on our table at 'Harmony' in Pretoria. That was a mistake! *A food apart.* We ate them with other foods, and the grape, more than any other fruit, is liable to fermentation. *It is chemically converted into poison when mixed with other substances in a perverted system.*

The stomach is nature's own laboratory. Put the right combinations of food into it, and the result is the fabrication of every essence necessary for life and health. But the stomach is also a still. At the temperature of blood-heat, the process of digestion is carried on in the form of fermentation. The manufacture of alcohol takes place. This seems to be indispensable to the well-being of the body, but an excess of alcohol causes a poisoning of the system. Toxaemia, or auto-intoxication (self-poisoning) takes place.

This is true when foods are mixed in the stomach indiscriminately, and especially so when to this mixture is added the grape. Taken into an impure stomach, it becomes a dangerous enemy. On the other hand, when by fasting, the system has been prepared for the change of diet, the grape becomes our greatest benefactor—our saviour from the ills of the flesh. In South Africa, in France and in Italy, and wherever the grape is largely used, cancer is as great a scourge as in any other part of the world. This is due to the wrong use of the fruit, and to ignorance of the dangers arising from an unscientific use of it.

The Grape is, as far as I know, the most powerful natural solvent of chemical deposits, and at the same time the most drastic eliminator. Because of its extraordinary properties, the avenues of excretion become superbly active under a proper grape cure. A volume could be dedicated to the remarkable effect of the grape on the nervous system."

Dr. Johanna Brandt's little book goes into approximately 30,000 words.

Here are other extracts:

"The patient should remember that every new ache and pain under the grape cure is an expression of life, of renewed activity. Nerves that have been atrophied for years have been stimulated by the grape. 'There is no pain.' Can this be said, truly, of a body of flesh and blood? I am afraid that deep spiritual teachings have been misapplied in our day. Physical pain is Mother Nature's own voice warning us of danger. She speaks through the nerves, those delicate, watchful and intelligent protectors of the human body. The point is of great importance in connection with the false doctrines of the day, especially in relation to chronic deafness, cataracts of the eye, goitres, diabetes and mental afflictions, in fact all so-called incurable diseases. The medical properties of the grape cannot be over-estimated. Salts of potash are found plentifully in grapes. . . . The grape is exceptionally rich in iron and is the finest natural tonic in the world."

Dr. Brandt writes on:

"The grape has vital relation to the proteid basis of the protoplasm of the cell and is on that account a quick repairer of tissue waste. As a flesh and muscle forming element it has no rival. The grape is a perfect food; almost without exception the most perfect food. Quite apart from its value as a solvent, it stands alone among the foods of nature as a body *builder*. I have administered it as a cure for tuberculosis and have witnessed the amazing spectacle of an emaciated patient putting on five pounds weight in one day, and three pounds the next, i.e. an increase of eight pounds in forty-eight hours. This took place after a fast of six or seven days. The grape is the most strengthening food. It is nourishing, sustaining and completely satisfying. Taken *without* salt or sugar, it cures all complaints of the stomach, bowels and liver, because of the abundance of natural salts and acids it contains. The organic acids of the grape are strongly antiseptic, and their effect on the gums is perhaps more valuable than any other result of the cure, for it means the preservation of the teeth on which mankind is dependent, not alone for health but for beauty. Would that I had the tongue of a Saint to warn you against the evil of having your teeth extracted because of poison at the roots; It is not always necessary. Every tooth may be loose in its socket, and pus may be pouring from the gums, but after a few weeks on the exclusive grape diet, you will find that the teeth are firmly set in the jaws, and that every trace of pyorrhoea poisoning has disappeared. *Try it. Prove it. Demonstrate the cure.*

There is said to be only one disease and that is blood disease. It is for the sake of convenience that we classify them into nervous, muscular, organic or constitutional diseases. As a matter of fact—barring accidents and malformations—we depend for life and health, solely on the condition of our blood. And our blood is dependent first on what we think; second on what we inhale, and third on what we eat and drink. To obtain control of these three essentials is to have perfect health. *Purifying the blood.* I am convinced that cancer is a blood disease, more so in fact than any other disease. No bruise could develop into cancer if the blood were pure, and so I say again most earnestly, give the grape cure a trial. Go to the root of the matter and remove the cause of the trouble. Or better still, prevent further trouble. There is nothing like the grape cure for purifying the blood from gouty and rheumatic poisons. The inorganic deposits that have settled between the joints are expelled in the form of diarrhoea, or more often, an unpleasant oily sweat. The loosening of the joints sometimes causes great pain, which may be relieved by poultices or compresses of fresh grape juice diluted with a little water. Pernicious anaemia may be cured by a pure grape diet. Appendicitis loses its terrors when the secret of the exclusive grape diet has been grasped. With the grape poultice on the affected part, the pain speedily subsides and the inflammation goes down.

The quickest cure. I used to think that fasting was the quickest cure we knew. But how much have I learned since 1925! There is no comparison between the fasting cure and the grape cure. Nothing can take the place of the complete fast in acute disease, but the fast only partially eliminates the inorganic deposits by which chronic diseases are caused. Perhaps that is the reason why cancer cannot be cured by fasting alone. One of the great and yet unsolved problems of medical science is how to establish in the diabetic and the goitre patient the normal sugar content of the blood.

Nature succeeds where science fails. A diet of raw fruits and vegetables corrects these abnormal conditions of the blood. But the grape cure is the quickest cure. The marvellously rapid action of the grape is due to the fact that the grape sugar is taken immediately into the circulation without undergoing any process of digestion. There is on that account no undue tax on the organs of digestion and assimilation, and Mother Nature can turn her full attention to the task of destroying the disease. The effect is sometimes instantaneous. But again I must remind the reader that this is *only true when grapes are taken alone and on a pure stomach.*

Unnatural cravings. The matchless grape is the supreme cure for the craving of alcoholic liquors. Supplying, as it does, the purest form of alcohol, which is indispensable to the maintenance of life and health, the grape should form the exclusive diet of our unfortunate fellow-creatures. It should be the only food used in our asylums, jails and penitentiaries; the only nourishment permitted in our hospitals before and after an operation. And in our homes every member of the family who is addicted to vice, to the drug habit, and to excessive use of tobacco, tea and coffee, should be persuaded to undergo a grape cure. Without compulsion or threat; the hapless victim of perverted appetite is eager to be liberated. A sane and simple way of achieving this appeals to him.

Sex problems. I see in this discovery of the grape cure the solution of sex and all other social problems. By the magical purification of the blood, the nerves are stabilised, self-control is established, and our God-given-heritage of sense and desire is transmuted into Divine creative power. No limit can be set to the stupendous importance of the grape cure. It is the most significant discovery of our age, because the physical well-being of the entire human race depends on it. And on this again depends spiritual unfoldment and the advance of science.

Emancipation. This means the emancipation of the world from the iniquities of war. Let us pause a moment here—try to picture this beautiful world in a state of peace. Not a negative peace. Thrilling with life and love, supremely active, charged with the magic power of confidence and strength.

Fearlessness. Emancipation from the horrors of the surgeon's knife, the dangers of the hypodermic use of morphia. The destruction of the nerves by the use of radium and electricity, and the complications arising from the introduction of poisonous inorganic medicines into the delicate human frame.

Material prosperity. Emancipation from financial care. The beautiful economy of the cure brings deliverance from the haunting fear of doctor's bills. The breadwinner can now begin to set aside some of his earnings for congenial purposes, or to make provision for his old age, instead of hospital expenses, chemists, druggists and dental bills. The cure can never be exploited for commercial purposes. There is no money in it. Our fruit growers alone will benefit from it.

Simplicity. And it is so simple that you can adopt it in your own home. It is only in extreme cases that patients are confined to their beds while undergoing the grape cure. To be able to go about one's work as usual is perhaps one of the greatest advantages of this cure. Think what it means to the business woman, the professional man, the University student!

Immunity. Power shall be added unto power. By the purification of the blood and the general upliftment of the mind and the body resulting therefrom, I see the peoples of the earth gradually becoming immune from disease. Germs, plagues and epidemics lose their terror. Fearlessness has been born. The entire mental outlook has been changed. Hopeful, constructive, optimistic, the sufferer sets about adjusting his faculties to this new psychology.

Children on the grape cure. Children who have been taught to fast when they feel out of sorts, have no difficulty in abstaining from food altogether. After a fast of two or three days, they go on the grape cure and are usually able to return to school at once. There have been no complications, very little time has been lost, and they resume their studies with minds clear and alert. In serious cases grape juice only should be administered. But what about the unfortunate child who has been taught to believe that he will die if he is not stuffed? A little strategy must be employed. Keep him in bed—out of doors in fine weather, and bring him a small bunch of grapes every two hours. Count the grapes and pop one into his mouth every minute, telling him to watch the hands of the clock himself, and to chew until it is time for the next grape. This is a great game. Children respond to the grape cure far more rapidly than adults. The dreaded operation for adenoids and tonsils is averted because the germ of disease is actually destroyed in the gums by the antiseptic properties of the grapes. This cure is the salvation of your children's teeth. Compare this with the destructive action of inorganic medicines on the teeth. Have you ever thought of the effect of medicine on the delicate lining of the throat and stomach after watching its effects on the hardest substance in the body—the enamel of the teeth?

Appeal. Reader, are you going to do your share towards checking the devastating tide of disease and premature death that is spreading over the globe? Then do not be satisfied when, after the grape cure, you have regained perfect health. Your own freedom from suffering is not enough. Think of the other members of the human family and pass the message on."